BEAUTY HACKS

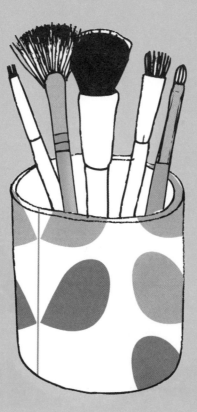

THIS IS A CARLTON BOOK

This edition published in 2016 by Carlton Books
An imprint of the Carlton Books Group
20 Mortimer Street
London W1T 3JW

First edition published in 2006
Second edition published in 2011

A CIP catalogue record for this book is available from the British Library.

ISBN 978 1 78097 705 8

Printed and bound in China

Illustrations: Sam Loman

This book reports information and opinions which may be of general
interest to the reader. It is advisory only and is not intended to serve as a
substitution for a consultation with a dermatologist, beauty therapist or
physician. Neither the author nor the publisher can accept responsibility
for any accident, injury or damage that results from using the ideas,
information or advice offered in this book.

The application and quality of beauty products, treatments, herbal
preparations and essential oils is beyond the control of the above parties
who cannot be held responsible for any problems resulting from their
use. Always follow the manufacturer's instructions. Do not use herbal
preparations or essential oils without prior consultation with a qualified
practitioner or medical doctor, if you are pregnant, taking any form of
medication or if you suffer from oversensitive skin.

BEAUTY HACKS

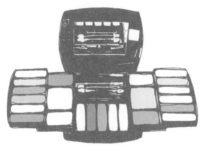

500
SIMPLE WAYS TO GORGEOUS SKIN, HAIR, MAKEUP AND NAILS

Esme Floyd

CARLTON
BOOKS

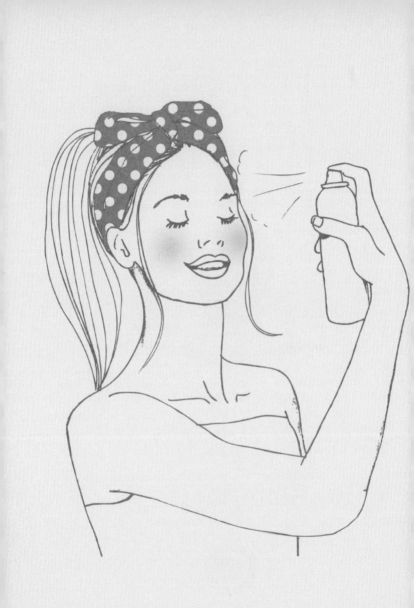

CONTENTS

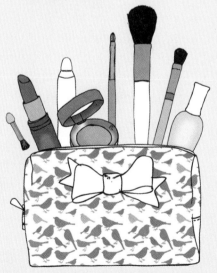

INTRODUCTION

Did you know that ketchup can help correct green tinges in blonde hair, that sun damage makes pores larger or that using a cool, bright lipstick colour will make your teeth look whiter?

Here we've gathered together 500 beauty hacks to help you get gorgeous from head to toe. Read through the categories that interest you or dip in and out to get quick, succinct advice for any beauty problem you face. From acne outbreaks to untidy eyebrows, from split ends to cellulite, you will find new techniques and solutions to help you improve the appearance and health of your body and let you put your best face forward every day.

TOP TEN BEAUTY HACKS

SKINCARE

ANTI-AGEING

BE ALERT TO BETACAROTENE

Betacarotene, a powerful natural anti-ageing antioxidant, is a pigment in yellow and red fresh foods that the body converts to vitamin A to generate new cells. Get your dose from apricots, peaches, nectarines, sweet potatoes, carrots and leafy greens.

SEEK OUT SELENIUM

Fish, red meat, chicken, grains and eggs contain selenium, an antioxidant which works with vitamin E against pollutants to combat skin ageing and cancer. Healthy sources include oil-rich nuts, seeds and avocados.

LOOK GREAT WITH GRAPES

Resveratrol, a polyphenol found in red grapes and an antioxidant and anti-cancer agent, helps mop up the damage caused by sun and pollution exposure, allowing the skin to help heal itself following damage. In addition to eating grapes, look for vinotherapy salon treatments and products that claim to harvest this ingredient.

STAY OUT OF THE SUN

Ninety per cent of problems associated with ageing are the result of too much sun exposure, so the best thing you can do to help your skin stay young is avoid the sun.

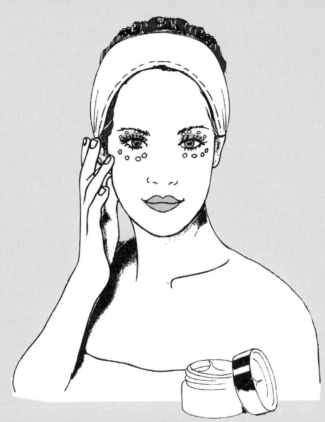

SMOOTH AWAY FINE LINES

To prevent ageing and ensure the delicate skin around your eyes
stays taut, apply an eye cream above and below the eye area
morning and night after the age of 25.

GET YOUR BEAUTY SLEEP

Sleep is one of the best ways to reduce the signs of ageing, by
allowing skin to replenish overnight. If you can't sleep, make
sure your room isn't too hot – the deepest sleep occurs if your
atmosphere is 18-24°C (64-75°F).

GIVE UP SMOKING

In smokers, skin looks sallow as a result of poor circulation and the action of drawing on the cigarette causes lines to be etched around the mouth. To reduce these signs of ageing, give up smoking if you're still doing it, and avoid smoky environments.

DRINK IT IN

Overall skin health depends on proper hydration, as the skin is the first organ to become dehydrated if you don't drink enough, causing sagging and lines. The optimum amount is 2.5 litres (5 pints) a day.

CLEANSING & CARE

BEWARE OF OVERCLEANSING

Overcleansing is a major cause of sensitive skin, as it strips the skin's underlayers of its natural protective properties. Make sure you use a cleanser that's right for your skin type and don't overdo it.

SLEEP CLEAN

It's an old adage, but never go to bed with your make-up on. It prevents the skin from shedding and breathing and may cause blemishes and/or blackheads to appear.

SPECIALIZE FOR EYES

For fast removal, use a good eye make-up remover rather than a cleanser. It has oils that dissolve make-up better and faster than regular cleanser or toner. Then wash as usual.

CLEANSE BEFORE YOU COLOUR

Before applying your make-up in the morning, make sure you thoroughly cleanse your face and apply moisturizer to even out the skin.

STEAM AWAY IMPURITIES

For a quick, deep cleanse, pour boiling water into a bowl with lemon juice and rose petals and hold your face over the bowl, covering your head with a towel. The steam will invigorate you, aid in respiration, and help loosen blackheads. Cleanse afterwards and follow with a cool-water rinse to close pores.

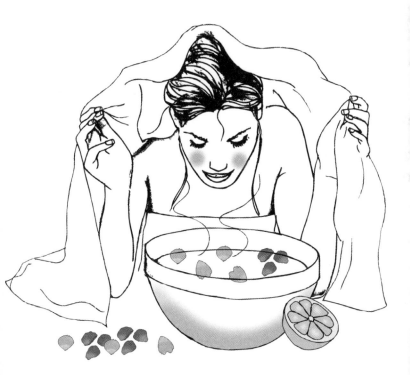

COSMECEUTICALS
& MIRACLE INGREDIENTS

GET SMOOTH WITH SOY

Soy proteins can help make skin temporarily smoother by
improving firmness and elasticity if applied regularly. Look for
them as ingredients in new hi-tech face creams.

GO MAD FOR MANGOSTIN

If you suffer from redness, blotchiness and broken capillaries on
the skin, look for Mangostin in your face cream. An extract from
the mangosteen fruit, Mangostin has been shown to help reduce
red patches, dark spots and other circulation-related troubles,
particularly when combined with antioxidant vitamins A, C and E.

C THE DIFFERENCE

Vitamin C (ascorbic acid) has a brightening effect on skin
as it helps boost circulation and collagen production, which
means skin looks and feels firmer and smoother as a result. It
is essential to the formation of collagen. Vitamin C is found in
high levels in citrus fruits, berries and kiwi, but also in serums,
creams and other beauty products.

CUCUMBER AND THYME

Cucumber and thyme contain anti-inflammatory and antiseptic
properties to soothe red, irritated skin, and are thought to be
especially powerful when used in combination with each other,
as they exert stronger effects.

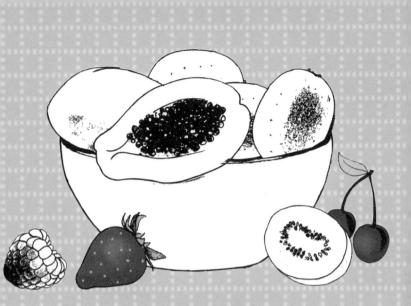

PAPAYA FOR PAPAIN ENZYME

Papaya contains the papain enzyme, a natural, nonabrasive botanical that dissolves dead skin cells, which makes it a great ingredient for face masks and exfoliators. It deep cleanses without stripping, leaving dull skin smoother and more refined.

LIGHTEN UP WITH LIQUORICE

Liquorice extract has been shown to have an evening and lightening effect on skin that will help fade age and sun spots if used over a few months. Many anti-ageing creams now contain it.

TAKE UP TOCOPHEROL

The ingredient alpha-tocopherol, found in face creams and sunscreens, is thought to optimize protection against damaging UVA and UVB rays, help prevent premature signs of ageing and stimulate collagen production to make the skin look younger.

SAY YES TO SAFFLOWER

Increasingly, cosmetic companies are waking up to the benefits of safflower oil to create and purify emulsions. The product increases the skin's absorption of oils without making it oily, so is a great choice for anti-ageing creams.

LOOK YOUNGER WITH MESOTHERAPY

Mesotherapy, in which vitamins, minerals and antioxidants are injected into the middle layer of the skin, is said to improve skin quality and vitality by replenishing the skin with essential vitamins that occur naturally within the cells. The vitamins A, E, C, D and B create firmness, clarity and smoothness in the skin.

REGENERATE WITH RETINOID

Retinoid is a vitamin A compound, available through pharmacies in the prescription Retin-A and in cosmeceuticals as retinol, which can help reduce fine lines and wrinkles by regenerating skin in the lower layers, sloughing off the upper layers and by stimulating collagen and elastin.

VITAMIN COCKTAILS

BioVityl and VitaNiacin technology is the newest way to give skin a vitamin boost, by combining vitamins the skin needs in one formula. The combination of vitamins cleverly increases absorption and makes the creams work better.

THINK ZINC

Zinc sulphate products like Cellex-C are naturally derived from plants and sometimes shellfish and have been claimed to have anti-ageing effects by smoothing the skin and protecting it from dehydration. It can help clear complexions prone to blemishes and can improve colour, tone and texture.

HYDROQUINONE FOR HYPERPIGMENTATION

Hydroquinone is a chemical ingredient in skin creams (and can appear under a wide range of brand names), which eases the appearance of patchy skin caused by hyperpigmentation. It is often delivered in a hyaluronic acid base to smooth the texture of skin further.

SAY HELLO TO HYALAURONIC ACID

Hyalauronic acid is a powerful ingredient that occurs naturally within our cells and contributes to the structural support of the skin if it soaks into the lower layers. Best used as a facemask or leave-on cream.

GIVE SKIN A FEAST

Skin is the last organ to get the benefits of the good things you eat, so often there's precious little nourishment left, even if your diet is fantastic. Choose face treatments high in essential minerals such as calcium, magnesium and zinc to give it a boost.

C FOR YOURSELF

Vitamin C is a natural skin protector, necessary for the formation of collagen. As an antioxidant it destroys harmful free-radicals in the body caused by pollution, stress and bad diet. Free radicals attack the skin, causing premature ageing, so vitamin C in creams and diet is a must.

CREAMS & SERUMS

DAY AND NIGHT
Always use separate day and night creams. The day creams are designed to absorb into the skin quickly and not interfere with make-up application whereas night creams are more emollient and designed for bare skin.

FIRM AND MOISTURIZE
For very dry or mature skin, a firming serum or treatment applied underneath a moisturizer gives an added boost.

TREAT COMBINED AREAS
A one-product moisturizer that contains AHAs should treat and normalize both dry and oily areas equally. There are also cleansers available with ingredients that leave dry areas moisturized and oily areas cleared of sebum.

DO IT SENSITIVELY
If you have easily reactive or sensitive skin, stick to simple, pure products without a cocktail of anti-ageing or AHA ingredients. These will simply replenish the natural moisture without triggering a problem.

PROTECT WITH UV
Always use a moisturizer with an SPF 15 to protect from sun damage. With modern formulations there is no need to apply both a sunscreen and a moisturizer.

DO IT DAILY WITH LIGHT MOISTURIZING

Every skin type needs a daily moisturizer, so know the one suitable for you. Lightweight gels and simple moisturizers are good for young and sensitive skins.

SERUMS ARE SERIOUSLY GOOD

Serums are pumps or vials of potent anti-ageing agents such as antioxidants and AHAs. Some are formulated for daily use under a moisturizer while others are for short-term or overnight use.

EXFOLIATORS & SCRUBS

EXFOLIATE FOR EXCEPTIONAL SKIN

If left on the body, dead skin cells flake, dry and peel quickly, so the best way to keep skin looking smooth, vital and evenly coloured is to scrub away those dead cells with a shower scrub.

BRUSH AND GO

If your lips are seriously dry or flaky, apply a little lip balm and brush them with a soft, dry toothbrush to boost circulation and remove all the dead skin cells while working the moisturizer into the deeper levels of your skin.

EXFOLIATE WITH CARE

Don't be tempted to rub too hard or use a too-grainy exfoliant on your face. Instead, choose small-grained products and keep it to once a week. If your skin looks red or patchy, you've gone too far.

SHIELD IN THE SUN

Newly exfoliated skin is more prone to sun damage, so apply a sun block after exfoliating if you're going to be exposed.

FACE FACTS WEEKLY

On your face, you should exfoliate once a week to remove dead skin cells. This will not only make your skin look fresher and more radiant, but also helps your products penetrate deeper into the epidermis, making them more effective.

STOP INGROWERS

Regular exfoliation has been shown to help prevent ingrown hairs and promote smoother skin as the skin 'gets used' to regenerating itself in response to the upper layers being removed efficiently.

DON'T MIX FACE AND BODY

Don't be tempted to use body exfoliators on facial skin, because products designed for the body are likely to be harsher and could be too abrasive for your face, resulting in irritation.

DON'T FORGET BUTTOCKS

It might not be the first thing people see about you, but don't neglect the skin of your buttocks, which can be prone to pimples and cellulite, if left untended. Use a bath mitt or puff to gently exfoliate in the bath or shower.

GO GENTLY

Overly vigorous exfoliating can break the tiny blood vessels under your skin, causing thread veins and redness to appear, especially on the delicate skin around the cheeks, eyes and neck. Be gentle and avoid exfoliators with natural grains, which are more abrasive than synthetics.

SKIN PROBLEMS

SCENT SENSITIVITY

Instead of using a scented sunscreen on sensitive skins, opt for an unscented alternative that contains organic, plant-based ingredients, such as aloe vera, jojoba, avocado and camomile.

PORES FOR THOUGHT

The best way to keep pores looking smaller and tighter is to keep them clean, washing your face twice a day – morning and evening – for best results with a mild cleanser.

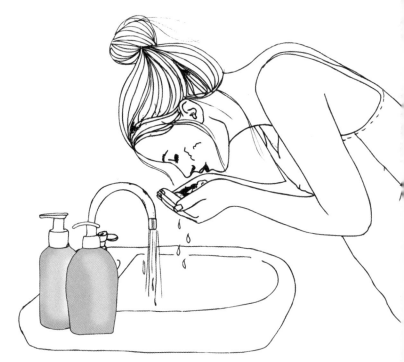

SPICE ISN'T NICE

Rosacea can be exacerbated by spicy foods containing chilli and mustard as well as hot drinks, which cause an increase in circulation and can make redness worse, as well as causing skin to feel hot and uncomfortable.

POLLUTION PROTECTION

Battle against polluted urban environments by using an SPF foundation or day cream specifically formulated to screen out the sun naturally with titanium dioxide, rather than one that contains chemicals, which will contribute to the overload of toxins and environmental chemicals.

EASE ECZEMA

The red, blistering itchy skin of eczema can be treated with a triceram cream, a nonsteroid with a ceramide base that helps the skin to repair. Balloon vine extract is an anti-inflammatory that can also help and is available in gel form.

IT'S HIP TO BE ROSE

For dry skin, choose products containing extract of rosehip. This ingredient contains high levels of omega-3 and omega-6 oils, which are nourishing for the skin. It also acts as an anti-inflammatory, which will soothe problem areas.

PEEL OFF THE LAYERS

You can now get similar results at home as you would from a medically administered chemical peel because of advances in technology. Over-the-counter 'peel' kits contain chemicals such as glycolic acid that dissolve the top layers of skin, lifting them off to reveal a brighter complexion. They usually have a two- or three-part process: the acid solution, an agent to calm the skin and stop the action and a moisturizer.

UNPLUG BLACKHEADS

One of the most effective ways to rid yourself of blackheads without damaging or bruising your skin is with pore-cleaning strips, available over the counter from most pharmacies. Because the skin isn't squeezed with this technique, it is not at risk from further infection.

ARREST PREMATURE AGEING

Rescue ageing skin by being scrupulous about using a sunscreen daily, keep out of the sun in summer and rescue early fine lines with intensive serums and brightening AHAs. You must use an SPF15 in combination with acids such as AHA and BHA.

HARSH PRODUCTS CAN HARM

If you suffer from rosacea, you should at all times avoid astringents and harsh soaps because not only can they make the symptoms worse, they also dry out skin, making it harder to treat and cover.

PIGMENT SKIN ALERT

If you are pregnant or suffer irregular skin pigmentation, avoid bergamot essential oil as this can cause uneven skin colour to become worse. Some concentrations are photo-toxic, and can accelerate pigmentation by making skin more sensitive to sunlight. Avoid exposure to the sun, sun lamps or tanning booths if using the oil.

PEROXIDE FOR PIMPLES

If you're prone to spotty breakouts, use a benzoyl peroxide solution on the affected area, which will dry out the area of oil and which also has antibacterial properties, which can help stop spots appearing.

WORK AWAY WHITEHEADS

If you suffer whiteheads, try applying a gel or cream containing salicylic acid to the pimple, a drying and toning agent which may help you to unplug the pores and prevent further outbreaks.

STEM THE ERUPTION

Cystic acne has the potential to leave deep scars so spots should never be squeezed. If it's an open pimple, apply an acne-drying gel or lotion and let it run its course. If you have frequent outbreaks, see a dermatologist.

HEAT IT UP

If you have to squeeze blackheads, apply a warm-to-hot flannel first to soften, then wrap a tissue around your fingers and gently squeeze. Never squeeze facial skin hard enough to leave an imprint.

FACIAL HARMONY

To improve red, itchy or allergic skins, visit a salon for a specific ultra-sensitive skin treatment. If plant-based products like arnica and cypress nut are used, they will reduce swelling and redness.

STEAM IT AWAY

It's almost impossible to prevent blackheads, but steam can help minimize them. Once a week, steam your face to soften the oils that clog the pores and follow with a deep-cleansing clay skin mask, rinsing thoroughly with warm water to clear the skin.

PREVENT SPREAD

If you're worried about infection from acne eruptions spreading to other parts of your face, use a topical antibiotic, which will help to contain the infection. Never squeeze, as it could make the pore swell further and look worse, and avoid metal extractor tools which can damage surrounding tissue.

HOLD THE SCRUB

Beware of over-exfoliating spotty or oily areas of the skin. On problem skin, exfoliation can cause excess oils to be released, making the problem worse, and it can cause acne to spread to uninfected areas. Instead, use gentle polishers to treat the oily areas only.

TONERS

BE ALCOHOL-FREE

Alcohol-based toners and cleansers are the enemy of dry skin, as they strip the skin dry of moisture and can cause problems with skin firmness and blemishes. If you suffer from dry skin, avoid products with alcohol and use a moisturizer more than once a day to keep skin plump and hydrated.

BE A T-ZONE SMOOTHIE

If you have combination skin, treat the different areas of your face independently – exfoliate the T-zone area, but leave cheeks alone, and when moisturizing concentrate on cheeks and neck, leaving only a light layer on the T-zone.

POUR COLD WATER ON IT

For a quick tone and boost for tired, dull skin, splash your face in cold water to bring fresh blood to the surface, stimulating circulation and giving you a healthy glow.

AVOID THE TINGLE

In general, products that make your skin tingle are too harsh – tingling in response to toners or cleansers is your skin's way of telling you to go for something weaker. Try toners that are designed for sensitive skin – look for those based on rosewater instead of witch hazel or alcohol.

WRINKLE-BUSTERS

KNOW YOUR WRINKLES

There are four different types of wrinkles – fine, deep, static and dynamic. Fine wrinkles, around the eyes, occur gradually due to the breakdown of collagen and elastin; deeper ones like forehead lines start in the muscles below the surface; dynamic lines are those seen only when your face moves; and static wrinkles are seen all the time.

REPAIR YOUR SKIN

Vitamin A can help diminish wrinkle depth, as its light inflammatory action 'puffs up' the skin so wrinkles look less deep. Find it in anti-wrinkle creams or add it to your diet by eating lots of fruit and vegetables.

WHITE AND GREEN TEA

Green and white tea can help delay collagen ageing and weakening, which has been shown to be a premier cause of wrinkles. Many face creams use green and white tea, not only for their anti-oxidant properties but also because white tea is shown to limit DNA damage in sun-exposed skin. White tea promotes new cell growth and strengthens the skin.

BE COOL IN SHADES

Sunglasses will stop lines developing around your eyes, caused by squinting against sun or harsh light. Problem areas are in cars and changes in light intensity between inside and outside. Wearing shades in winter, when the sun is lower, is important, too.

WITCH HAZEL FACE FIRMER

Witch hazel can temporarily tighten the skin and give facial tissues a lift. Instead of using it neat, which can stress delicate skin, mix 1 teaspoon with 100g (3½ oz) of moisturizer and after two weeks you should see results.

SILK SIREN

For the smoothest facial skin, copy the Egyptian queens and insist on a silk or satin pillow, which will smooth out facial wrinkles while you sleep and ensure you wake up looking your best.

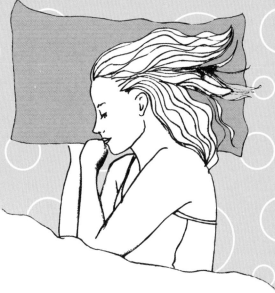

THE FACE

BASE-IC RIGHTS

PAT IT OFF

After your make-up application, use a soft tissue to gently pat over your face. This will blend the make-up together and soften the look to help you appear natural without leaving you with uncovered patches.

DON'T CREASE UP

Applying eye creams and moisturizers before foundation lessens the probability of creasing because it smoothes out lines in the delicate under-eye area.

DITCH A DOUBLE CHIN

Get rid of your double chin by using a slightly darker shade of powder or foundation under your chin, which will make it appear to recede. Blend towards the back of the jawline to add definition.

TONE UP

Always choose a foundation that blends with your natural skin tone and never try to counteract your skin colour with a cosmetic. Asian skins have an underlying golden base so you need to choose yellow-based options. Ruddy complexions are best with ivory- or pink-based shades.

AVOID THE GREY FOR DARK SKINS

Too many foundations for dark and black skins are chalky and ashen. To find the right shade, look for rich colours in a sheer formulation that will allow your natural skin colour to shine through, while evening out pigmentation. Very matt formulas are the worst culprits for a greyish cast.

GO OIL-FREE

In warm, humid weather, skin is prone to producing more oil. Therefore the first port-of-call when summer comes round is an oil-free foundation. Oil-free liquid and sheer formulations are good matt, lightweight options that won't clog pores or leave shine.

LIKE LIQUID FOR DAY

For the sort of sheer-to-medium coverage that looks great in the daytime, try liquid foundations. These spread on easily and will last all day without becoming heavy or settling into fine lines. Always shake the bottle gently first to distribute the contents and apply to the centre of the face using light, dabbing movements with the finger-tips before gently blending outwards.

A WHITER SHADE OF PALE

If you prefer a pale, porcelain face with a flawless finish, use a white-coloured skin primer to give an all-over, even base before you apply a foundation. The primer will help avoid the need for touch-ups.

BEWARE OF FACIAL HAIR

Try to avoid using thick foundations or powder on areas where you have facial hair. These products can cause the hairs to become more visible by forming a coating over them. If coverage is essential, wipe off any excess with a tissue.

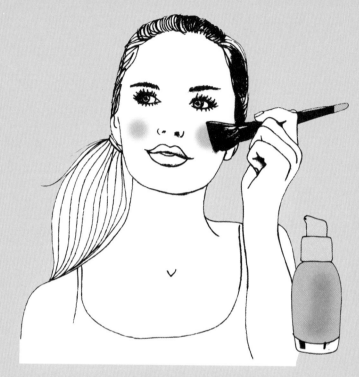

GET PUMP ACTION

If you can, choose a foundation in a tube or pump dispenser. These are good because the product can't slip back into the container after it has been exposed to air or touched, thus reducing the risk of contamination.

LONG FOR LONGLASTING?

A cream-to-powder foundation formula is a good option for dry and mature skins. It goes on as a rich, creamy moisturizer, but dries to a matt velvety finish that looks immaculate and provides good, long-lasting coverage, which won't 'slip' or rub off during the day like many cream-based foundations.

USE AN INSTANT MIX

For a lighter look in seconds, mix your foundation with your daily moisturizer in the palm of your hand before applying it. This homemade, tinted moisturizer will give you a light, even coverage and is a perfect solution for summer months when you want a lighter weight of formula.

BRONZE AWAY REDS

If you have a ruddy complexion or uneven, browny-red skin tones, think about using a beige foundation or a bronzer to maintain the natural look while evening out skin tone. Many very pale foundations have a pinky undertone that will exacerbate redness.

NEUTRALIZE YELLOW

Get rid of yellow skin tones, especially in sallow skin around the eyes, using a violet skin correction colour.

BLEND, BLEND, BLEND

After you have applied your foundation, make sure you spend a few minutes blending it onto your jawline, hairline and slightly onto your neck. Spend twice as long on your foundation as you do on any other element of your make-up.

FORGET YOUR LINES

If you have lines on your forehead, apply a light, oil-based foundation and set with a little translucent, light reflective powder to hide the lines away.

CREAMY CHEEKS

If the skin on your cheeks is dry, go for a creamy or oil-based foundation that will help smooth out dry skin and stop make-up flaking and peeling. Moisturize first for best results.

OPEN WIDE

When applying foundation, open your mouth to expose the neck area and allow you to blend your base over the jawline, to avoid an obvious line. Alternatively do it afterwards to check you've blended properly.

LOOK FRESH AS A DAISY

Freshen foundation at the end of the day by dabbing moisturizer under the eyes and smoothing it across the cheekbones for a touch of added sheen.

SPF IS ESSENTIAL

If you are not using a moisturizer with a SPF, make sure your foundation contains one – it is not necessary for both to have an SPF as you won't get increased protection.

BROWS

SHAPELY BROWS

To determine exactly where your brow should begin, imagine a vertical line or hold a make-up pencil straight alongside one nostril. Where the pencil lands by your brow is where it should begin. To work out where the brow should end, imagine a line from the outside of your nostril to the outer corner of your eye, extending out to your brow.

THREAD IT AWAY

Threading is a form of hair removal. It uses a small thread that is twisted around the eyebrow hairs to pull them out by the root. It is recommended for eyebrow shaping because it's less painful and not as harsh on the delicate skin than hot waxes.

DEFINE WITH A PENCIL

Pencils give the cleanest, most precise definition, but beware of drawing long lines. Instead, use light, feathery strokes to mimic hair growth.

GO TO A PROFESSIONAL

Take the easy route to perfect eyebrows by having your brows shaped by a beautician the first time you try re-shaping. All you then have to do is keep to the lines she's created for you, which takes much less time (and risk).

DIVIDE BY FOUR

For the best shape, think geometrically, as if the brow is divided into four sections along the length of the eye. The first three should head upward and the outer quarter should slant down.

KEEP BROWS IN LINE

If you want your eyebrows to stay in place, add a coat of clear mascara or a little hairspray on the eyebrow groomer before brushing to the desired shape.

COMB IT UP

Comb brows upward before plucking or colouring in to make sure you preserve the natural browline. If your brows are very thick or long, trim the hairs that extend above the upper line of the arch.

POWDER IT RIGHT

Eyebrow powder should be one to two shades lighter than your hair colour. A matching colour to your hair can look overpowering on a face and anything much darker is just too severe.

KEEP IT SHARP

Sharpen your eyebrow pencil before every application to make sure you keep the high definition look you're after. You can always blend if lines are too sharp.

CATCH THE HIGHLIGHTS

To make brows appear higher and more defined, apply some highlighting powder or cream under the middle to outer edge of the eyebrow, which will add fullness to the eye area.

GET SHEEN WITH VASELINE

Tame wayward eyebrow hairs with a tiny amount of brow fixative or Vaseline after you've applied your brow colour. This will give them a bit of added shine as well as holding them in place.

POWDER AND PEAK

Powders give a soft effect and need minimal blending. To heighten the arch, apply an extra bit of colour at the highest peak to make it stand out.

ENHANCE YOUR ARCHES

If you have a natural arch, work with it rather than creating a new one. If you need to create an arch, look into your eyes. The top arch of your eyebrow should fall directly above the outside of your iris for eye-opening results.

COLOURING IN

If you want to reshape your eyebrows, but are worried about making a mistake, fill in the area you want to preserve using an eyebrow pencil and pluck outside the edges. This way you won't over-pluck and you can perfect the shape first.

BRUSH THOSE BROWS

An old toothbrush is excellent for brushing brows after
pencilling in. Not only will it smooth down hairs, it will also
soften pencil lines, leaving them looking more natural.

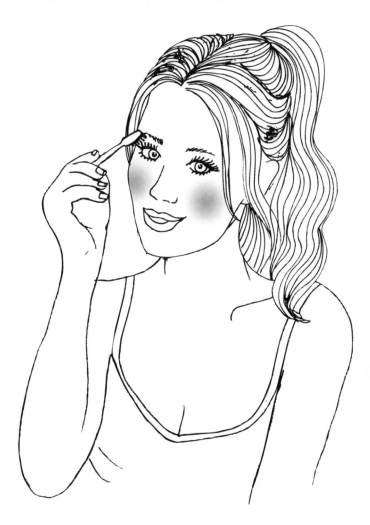

CHEEKS

GIVE YOURSELF A SMILE
To make blusher pay, smile into the mirror to find the apples of your cheeks, then brush the colour there in wide, sweeping movements for a natural, cheeky glow.

KEEP TO THE CURVE
Never apply blusher right up to the hairline, which is a sure fire way to make your face look unnaturally painted. Stop on the top curve of your cheekbone.

DARKEN FOR DEFINITION
To bring out your natural cheekbones, use a medium beige blush underneath to help the bones stand out – avoid dark colours or you will get a stripy look.

DON'T FREAK OVER STREAKS
If your blusher looks streaky or stripy, or if you have over coloured, don't be tempted to add more colour to even out the stripe. The only way to deal with it is to remove some colour with a tissue and dust a little translucent powder over cheeks.

LEAVE IT TILL LAST
For super-smooth results with no streaking, particularly for evening looks, apply blusher after powder. This will form a smooth, natural base that the colour can cling to.

CREATE CHEEKBONES

Cheekbones are best defined with highlighter rather than blusher, which can cause overcolouring. Blend a line of highlighter along the top edges of your cheekbones and a line of shade underneath to help them stand to attention.

GET IT RIGHT ON YOUR WRIST

Look for the most natural blush colour you can find. Try it on the inside of your wrist when choosing – if it looks natural here, it will look natural on your cheeks.

TWO WILL DO

Never go more than two shades darker than your natural skin tone. Bronzers are meant to warm your skin as if you have a natural glow, rather than adding colour.

HOW TO DO DEWY

Powder bronzers are best for oily complexions. If your skin is dry or you like a dewy finish, choose a cream, stick or gel to achieve your colour.

BLUSH IT UP

For lighter complexions, use a small amount of bronze on your cheeks and forehead. Follow this with a touch of pink or rose blush on the apples of your cheeks, for a natural-looking flush.

FINGER PAINTING

Cream, stick and liquid bronzers should be applied using your fingers. Dab them onto the apples of your cheeks and blend, using circular motions, toward the hairline. Leftover colour can be very lightly dabbed onto the bridge of the nose, on the temples and even on the collarbone.

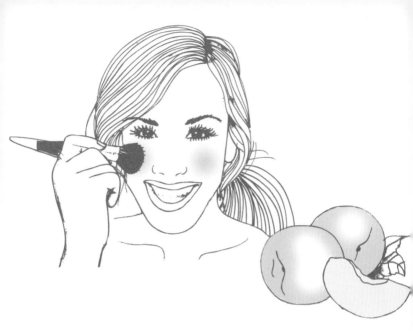

BE A PEACH BABE

Choose soft natural pinks, beiges and tawny peaches for daytime. These will blend with the tones in natural daylight and avoid making you look overdone. Go brighter and cooler at night for definition.

CONCEAL IT

DON'T GO TOO LIGHT

The most common mistake women make when applying concealer is choosing a colour that is too light. This merely achieves the opposite effect by actually highlighting the problem, especially if you're using it to cover under-eye circles.

CONCEAL DARK CIRCLES

Concealer is the most important step in banishing dark circles
and preparing the skin for a perfectly even base. Gently pat a
light reflecting creamy concealer above and below the eye area
to disguise imperfections. Avoid powdery sticks that can pull the
skin.

STICK IT TO LAST

Stick concealer lasts the longest of any type because it's less
prone to drying out or discolouring over time. Liquid-based
concealers may start to separate or go lumpy when they're past
their date.

COVER IT UP WITH GOLD

For concealing under-eye circles, which can often appear bluish
in colour, choose a gold-based, warm-toned concealer that will
counteract the blue and help you hide them.

COVER YOUR EYES

If you're covering up under-eye circles, don't just put the
concealer under the eye, which can give you a 'striped' look.
Instead, cover the whole eye area and set with a light dusting of
powder.

CONCEAL ALL DAY

Apply foundation before camouflaging problem areas with a
cream concealer. Finally, dot with translucent powder to hold the
concealer in place all day long.

EYE CARE

HORSE AROUND

For reducing under-eye bags, creams containing vitamin K and horse chestnut are thought to exert beneficial effects by reducing puffiness and blood flow under the thin skin of the area.

GO GENTLY INTO THE NIGHT

When you apply night cream under your eyes, do so gently. Use your fourth finger (which is the weakest) and pat the cream back and forth under the eye, starting at the outer corner and working inward.

SOOTHE EYES WITH CUCUMBER

Place a slice of cucumber on each eyelid for 10–15 minutes to allow the high water and mineral content of the cucumber to be absorbed into your delicate eye skin.

EYELINER

WIDEN WITH WHITE

To give your eyes the appearance of being wider set, line the inside of the bottom rim of your eyes with a soft white eyeliner pencil. This will also give you a fresher, younger look.

STAY OUTSIDE

Unless you're blessed with almond-shaped eyes, stick to using eyeliner on the outside rather than inside the lash line. Applying it inside will make your peepers seem smaller and dull their colour.

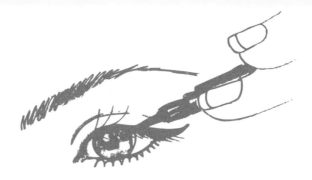

KEEP LIQUID THIN

Liquid eyeliners are great for a defined evening look, but don't extend the line beyond the natural corner of the eye and keep it thin for the most glamorous look. If you have trouble keeping steady, try making three dashes – at the inner, middle and outer corners, then joining them up.

DON'T BE BLUNT

Sharpen your eye pencil every time you use it. This prevents eye bacteria building up on the round, blunt end, which could spread to other parts of your eyes. It will also help you achieve high definition as blunt ends are much harder to control.

MODERNIZE YOUR EYES

Instead of using eyeliner for daily make-up, use powder eyeshadow applied with a very narrow brush to give a smokey, modern appearance to the edge of eyes. Smudge further if necessary with a larger brush. Alternatively, use the powder wet for a sharper line of colour.

HIDE EYE CIRCLES

To draw attention away from under-eye bags or circles, avoid applying eyeliner or mascara to lower lashes, which could draw attention downward instead of up.

EYESHADOW

COMPLEMENT, DON'T COLOUR

The purpose of eyeshadow is to shape and accentuate the eye, not colour it. Even if you're going bright, choose tones that accentuate your natural shades.

GET BRAND SAVVY

If you're using two shades of powdered eyeshadow, use the same brand, as they are more likely to be of the same formula, thus easier to blend with each other.

LINE UP THE BROWN

For paler skins, light browns and taupe eyeliners work best because they enhance the natural tones of the eye without overpowering the surrounding skin.

BE A ONE-TRICK WONDER

As a general rule, let your eyes or your lips do the talking – not both. This doesn't mean neglecting either area, just plump for a more natural look for one and use stronger make-up on the other. Usually you will want to concentrate on your best feature.

LONG MAY IT LAST

If you want your eyeshadow to last all day, prime your eyelids with a thin layer of foundation before applying your eye colour. If you forgo shadow for a bare look, it will also help your eyelids blend in with the skin tone on the rest of your face, in which case using mascara will be necessary to give your eyes some definition.

KEEP IT NEUTRAL

Do use flattering neutrals to contour and highlight your eyes for a timeless daytime look that will last. For eyeliners, stick to classic colours like black, navy or brown.

TOUCH IT UP

If you're in a hurry, add extra touches of cream or gel-type eyeshadow with the tip of your middle finger. Just a dot of the product, applied lightly, should work just fine.

GLOW FOR GOLD

Give eyes a gorgeous glistening glow for summer by dusting a shimmer golden bronzer or loose gold dust over eyelids and cheekbones. To add intensity, highlight the outer corners of your eyes with a darker copper or brown eyeshadow.

CREAMS INCREASE CREASES

Lightly powder lids before eyeshadow to keep them crease-proof longer. If you're prone to creasing, avoid cream colours in favour of silky powders.

FOIL SPILLS

Apply a dusting of loose powder directly under-eye area before you apply your eyeshadow. Afterwards, whisk away the powder from under your eyes with a brush and it will take eyeshadow fallout with it.

BRING EYES OUT WITH LIGHT

On deep-set eyes, choose shadow colours that are on the light side of the colour spectrum, particularly on the bit of lid directly above the eye, which will make them appear more prominent.

FACE MASKS

GO EASY FOR SENSITIVE SKIN

If you find your skin reacts badly to masks, but you still want to use them, try those with gentler ingredients like camomile and cucumber, and avoid lanolin, which can often cause reactions.

BE A SMOOTH-SKINNED HONEY

Honey and almond flour, mixed together into a paste, is an excellent scrub for oily skin because of honey's antiseptic properties and the high levels of vitamins they both contain. Its graininess makes it an excellent gentle exfoliator.

POST-MASK MOISTURE BOOST

Always moisturize directly after using a mask, unless the mask is a leave-on product and you are instructed to rub in the residue. With dead skin cells sloughed off and pores unclogged, your moisturizer will sink in more deeply and have greater penetrating results.

CLEANSE BEFORE YOU COVER

You wouldn't polish a dirty floor and neither should you put a mask on a dirty face. You'll only get the full benefits if you apply the mask to cleansed skin, which will allow your face to absorb more of the ingredients in the mask.

MIX UP A VITAMIN BLEND

Create a replenishing face mask with the flesh of one avocado, a little orange juice, honey, molasses and a few drops of camomile essential oil whizzed together in a blender to give your skin a vitamin boost.

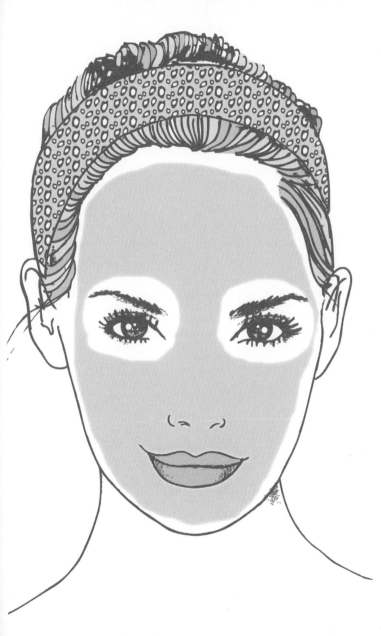

43

FINISH WELL

If you didn't exfoliate before a mask, finish by removing the mask using a warm, wet face cloth in gentle circular movements. This will act as a gentle exfoliant and leave skin instantly brighter and clearer-looking. However do not use a scrub or product exfoliator at this stage as you do not want to strip the skin.

BREW UP A STORM

For oily skin, a brewer's yeast mask can help tone without drying out. Mix a teaspoon of brewer's yeast with enough natural yogurt to make a loose, thin mixture. Pat this thoroughly into the oily areas and allow it to dry on the skin. After 15–20 minutes, rinse off with warm water, then cool and blot dry.

GO GENTLY WITH CUCUMBER

For gentle rehydration for sensitive skins, combine half a cucumber, scooped out of its skin, one tablespoon of yogurt, a few strawberries, and one teaspoon of honey. Apply to your face and allow to dry, then gently wipe off.

HIT BLEMISHES WITH A CARROT STICK

A carrot mask can work wonders for blemished complexions. Use a small, raw carrot mashed to a smooth paste or boil one in a little water and mash it. Then pat the mask all over the blemished areas and leave on for 15–20 minutes. Rinse and pat dry.

LAY IT ON THICK

Masks work best when coverage is generous, so don't be afraid to use a thicker application. This is one case when trying to skimp is a false economy because the mask won't do as much for the skin if it's thin and you'll only be more tempted to use it more often.

HIGHLIGHTERS

DON'T SWEAT IT

Illuminators and highlighters are great for picking out areas you want to highlight, but take care when applying them as a skin base or you could end up looking as if you have a sweaty face. Mix a tiny amount with your usual foundation for best results.

BE A RADIANT WOMAN

A perfect remedy for hungover skin, radiance boosters are applied after moisturizer and before foundation, but they also work well when patted over make-up for a quick, mid-day perk-up. They add instant glow, making you appear more wide-awake and fresher.

BOOST WITH A SPRITZ

Spritzing rosewater or a water spray over make-up is an instant reviver. It rehydrates skin and adds a natural glow, helping to get that natural dewy look without adding any extra product.

GOLDEN GIRLS

Gold-based highlighters are great in the summer when applied on top of bare skin or for darker complexions. In the cooler winter light, however, choose the pink versions that will give the same effect.

LIPS

PLUMP UP YOUR LIPS

Newly developed lip plumping glosses, with swelling ingredients like cinnamon and menthol, claim to temporarily inflate the pout, mimicking the effects of permanent surgical lip fillers like collagen and hyalauronic acid.

PEAK A POUT

Instead of completely outlining the lips, for a bigger pout just pencil in the cupid's bow, the centre of the bottom lip, and the corners of the mouth with a natural shade. This will enhance the shape of your lips, bringing attention to the edges and giving them a fuller appearance.

GET FLAWLESS COLOUR

To achieve the exact colour of the lipstick on your lips, apply a nude lip pencil to your lips before the lipstick. It will also help keep the lipstick in place for longer and reduce the chances of smudging.

STRIVE FOR EQUALITY

If you have a thinner top lip, you can help it stand out more by applying a slick of gloss to the top lip only to accentuate it, then blotting gently onto the lower lip.

KEEP LIPSTICK OFF YOUR TEETH!

Once you've applied your lipstick, put your forefinger in your mouth and then (just like a lollipop) slowly pull it out. All the lipstick that would have ended up on your teeth will have been successfully removed and you will be able to smile with security.

GET LUSCIOUS LIPS

Just as your face needs regular moisturizing, so too do your lips. Before you go to bed is the perfect time to really allow the moisture to sink in. Before you go to sleep, apply a large dose of your favourite lip balm and wake up in the morning with a perfectly rehydrated pout.

SEAL IT WITH AN E

To seal in lipstick instantly, prick a vitamin E capsule and slick it over your lip colour.

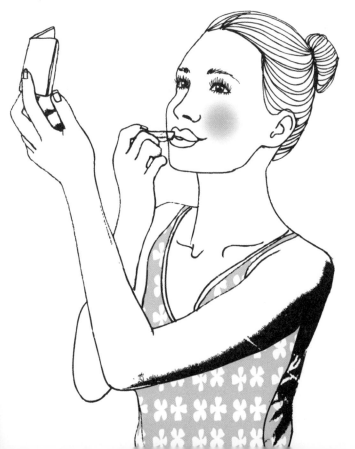

FIGHT FEATHERING

To prevent lipstick from feathering, line your mouth with a lip pencil, which will fill in lines and help to keep colour intact.

MAKE SURE YOU MATCH

Always choose a lipliner that matches your lip colour, then if your lipstick wears off you won't look overdone.

BE A GOOD CHAP

Use a Chapstick as a lip primer under colour. The waxiness smoothes the lip surface, fills tiny lines and will help hold the colour for longer. This is particularly useful under matt colours, which can add to the appearance of dryness.

TOUCH BASE WITH YOUR LIPSTICK

To form a perfect lipstick base, apply a light covering of foundation with a wet sponge and allow to dry. This will even out underlying skin tone and allow lipstick to stay on for longer.

BE A GLOSS LEADER

Create fullness with a spot of gloss in the middle of the mouth, particularly on the upper lips, which will appear fuller as a result.

DON'T BE SHY OF BIG LIPS

If your lips are large, don't be shy; promote them as a star feature using a deep coloured, matt lipstick. Avoid gloss and really bright colours, which can overly increase the voluptuous effect.

SAY IT BRIGHT

Lightweight brightening creams can give thin lips a natural-looking pout if blended over the lip line before using lipstick or gloss.

GO THE EXTRA SMILE

Make your lips look fuller by using a pale or frosty lipstick and finish with a splash of gloss in the middle of your mouth to achieve the perfect pout.

MASCARA

WEAR LIGHT LAYERS

Three or four coats of thinly applied mascara are more alluring and natural-looking than one or two clumpy applications. When it comes to eyelashes, the thinner the better!

GO WIDE

Concentrate mascara application on the outside of the eye – this will help to widen eyes and bring attention to the curved edges, making them appear more alluring.

MIRROR YOUR MASCARA

To apply mascara easily, look down into a mirror and brush through lashes from roots to tips, first on top then on the underneath of lashes. This will help avoid the brush hitting the eyelid.

ONE COAT AT A TIME

Apply one coat of mascara carefully and wait for it to dry before considering a second one. You may only need one application, this way, you'll avoid clogging.

LUBRICATE YOUR LASHES

Rub Vaseline, baby oil or eyelash conditioner into eyelashes overnight (do this with your eyes closed). This will help keep your lashes conditioned and prevent any breakage of the ends.

WARM UP MASCARA

If your mascara thickens when it reaches the end of the tube, place the sealed tube in warm water for a few minutes to help make the mascara thinner.

TRIM YOUR FALSIES

Trim false eyelashes before you apply them to mimic the natural shape of your eyelashes and to define your eyes. Make the outer edges longer for eye-widening results.

GET BEDROOM EYES

False lashes have improved dramatically and salons now offer extensions that can last up to three months. They are glued on lash by lash and offer fantastic length and colour, but you must follow strict care guidelines.

BRUSH AWAY CLOGS

If you don't have a mascara comb to hand, get rid of nasty looking clogs by following your mascara application with a quick brush through with an old, washed-and-dried mascara wand.

GET THE WIGGLES

When applying mascara, wiggle your wand on the base of the lashes. It's the mascara near the roots – not the tips – that gives the illusion of length and thickness.

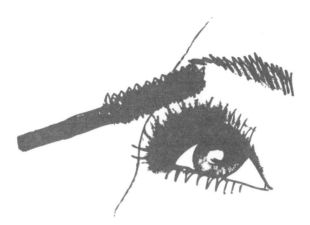

WASH BEFORE THE WAND

Always wash your hands before applying mascara to cut down the risk of passing on bacteria with your hands, especially if you're one of those people who uses their hands to touch their eye area while they apply.

WORK THE WAND

First, apply mascara to the middle and inner lashes using upward strokes, then concentrate on the outer lashes, sweeping out at a 45-degree angle to enhance the outer edge of the eye.

KINKS AND CURLS

Nothing opens up eyes more than curling the eyelashes. Curl at the base first, then at the halfway point to finish. Hold for about ten seconds, and always curl on clean lashes. Heat a metal curler under a hot hairdryer for a few seconds first to replicate the effects of a heated eyelash curler.

PERFECT SMILE

GET INTERDENTAL
If you have gappy teeth, bridges or implants, an interdental brush is often better than floss for cleaning between the teeth and keeping gums in the pink.

CHOOSE CHLORHEXIDINE
Chlorhexidine is the best ingredient to beat inflamed gums or gum disease. It is designed for short-term use and is available in special mouthwashes.

DISCLOSE YOUR WEAKNESS
Two-thirds of people who brush their teeth twice a day leave plaque deposits behind. Chew a disclosing tablet after brushing and any remaining plaque will turn red, enabling you to spot and target your trouble spots.

SCRAPE YOUR TONGUE
Tongue scraping is a very important part of oral hygiene as it rids the mouth of bacteria that can lead to bad breath and plaque build-up that can also stain the teeth.

JOIN THE JET-SET
Dental water jets are designed to be used after flossing for additional cleaning and polishing. They can be useful for people with bridges, implants or gum disease.

SHIFT STAINS WITH STRAWBERRIES

A simple, natural way to brighten teeth and get rid of stains is to cut a strawberry in half and run the juicy surface along your teeth.

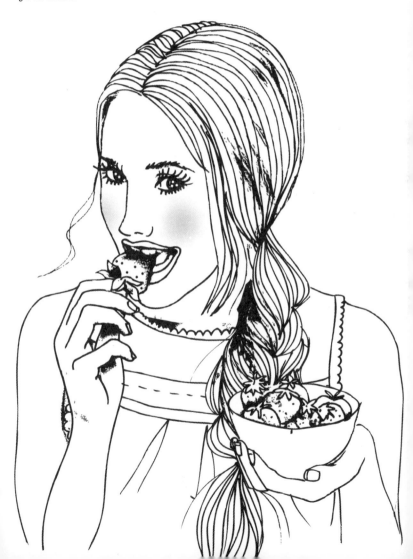

GUM MASSAGE

Dentists recommend gentle gum massage to strengthen and firm gums, enhance blood flow to the area, fight gingivitis and prevent disease. You can use special gum brushes for this purpose, or massage the gums daily with your index finger – combine with a herbal gum wash or oil for added benefit.

INVEST IN LEMON ZEST

Whiten teeth naturally by brushing with grated lemon zest, a natural bleaching agent that will whiten teeth without damaging your gums.

HOME TEETH WHITENING

Whiten your teeth at home with an over-the-counter gel and tooth tray. You will need to use this for several hours in the day or overnight and should see the maximum results in two or three weeks.

LASER AWAY STAINS

A bleaching system that uses a laser and a whitening gel is a one-off treatment that gets quick, immediate results. A laser light activates the gel and penetrates the enamel.

TOOLS OF THE TRADE

LIGHT IT UP

If you have a habit of overdoing your make-up, make sure you're using a mirror with a powerful enough light. Overdone cheeks or foundation 'tide marks' are common mistakes for people who lack voltage.

SIZE IT UP

For the most effective application, choose make-up brushes that match the size of the area they are to be used on. Brushes for eyelids will be smaller than cheek brushes.

LOOK WHERE YOU'RE GOING

Low-level-lighting can completely alter a look. Whatever light you're going to be seen in, try to make-up in a similar light or at least take the time to check how your make-up looks in similar conditions. To avoid mistakes use a make-up mirror that has several light options for day and night and cool and warm lighting.

LAY A GOOD FOUNDATION

Foundation applied with a sponge is a great choice for everyday make-up as it is literally painted onto the skin. The sponge allows you to build-up layers, which means you can start with a thin layer and go thicker for problem areas.

VIVE LA DIFFERENCE

There is nothing more frustrating than trying to apply a light shade and getting a darker smudge as a result of the last colour you used with the same brush. Keep brushes for dark and light shades separate.

FLUFF YOUR LINES

Invest in a large, fluffy brush for applying cheek colour – this will ensure soft, natural-looking lines when you apply it.

MILD BENEFIT

To avoid irritation, use a daily cleanser or a mild washing-up liquid to wash your brushes. These are more gentle alternatives to the specially formulated brush cleaners that can be harsh and cause skin reactions.

CULL YOUR MAKE-UP BAG

Make-up might rarely come with use-by dates, but often it's just like food – leave it too long and it will go off. Don't keep lipsticks for more than two years, foundation for more than a year or sunscreen for more than six months to be super-safe.

WASH THOROUGHLY

Wash your make-up brushes in soapy water at least every three months to keep them clean and clog-free. If someone else uses your brushes, wash them thoroughly before you use them again or you risk introducing bacteria into your make-up. Cosmetic sponges and applicators should be washed once a week. Rinse them well and dry flat.

GET BACK IN SHAPE

Reshape your brushes after washing, laying them out flat and letting them dry naturally before reusing them. If the bristles frizz and shed, it's time to buy new ones as there's no way to recondition the brushes once they are worn out. Keep an eye on the shape, too – each brush has a specific shape for an application purpose and once this deteriorates you will not get good results.

HAIRCARE

COLOUR

A CAP FOR BLONDES

If you have bleached or naturally blonde hair, avoid chlorine, which can make your hair turn green. Cover up with a swimming hat or use anti-chlorine shampoo to keep your colour looking natural.

CARROT JUICE FOR REDHEADS

If you're an orange tone redhead, enhance your natural colour with carrot juice left on the hair for five minutes and shampooed out as normal. The carrot pigment will boost the orange tones and leave your hair looking thick and colour conditioned.

BEET UP YOUR RED

For a great post-shampoo colour rinse for red-toned hair, infuse a chopped beetroot in hot water for ten minutes and use the water to rinse clean hair through to boost the natural red tones of hair and add depth and richness to colour.

GET RICH WITH ROSEMARY

To make the most of hair colour, add richness to brunette hair by infusing rosemary in hot water for ten minutes and allow to cool until warm. After shampooing, rinse through with infused water, followed by a small cold-water rinse to add shine.

COLOUR BLONDE WITH CAMOMILE

A great way to enhance shine and colour in blonde hair is to use cool camomile tea as a rinse following hair washing. This coats the hair and allows the natural blondeness to come through without product build-up.

CAMOUFLAGE GREY HAIRS

Older hair takes colour less well than young hair and skin. Instead of an all-over block colour, try highlights or lowlights, which give hair a sun-kissed appearance without appearing unnatural.

DO THE DIRTY

Don't turn up at the hair salon for a recolour with freshly washed hair. Roots show up better on unwashed hair, which is also easier to handle.

BE A RINSE PRINCESS

Instead of trying to dye your hair at home, which can lead to unnatural looking results, use a conditioning colour rinse, which will highlight natural colour and help boost the condition of hair as well.

VEG OUT THE GREY

The best way to cover grey hair is to opt for a shade lighter than your own in a natural vegetable dye, which will colour the hair naturally without drying or causing damage.

CUT TO SHAPE

SEE AN EXPERT

The number one tip for great hair is to get a good haircut. They can be expensive, but you're likely to recoup all the money you've spent on a quality professional because you'll need far fewer products (and time) to make it look good once you get home. The style will keep its shape for longer, too.

SQUARE UP TO SOFT LAYERS

If you have a square-shaped face, steer clear of bobs or short styles that accentuate your strong jawline. Instead, go for softer layers around the face to break up and cut into the squareness, and bring more attention to eyes and forehead.

LAYER IT OVAL

Oval faces are the most versatile face shape for styles. They do, however, work best with layers, long or short, which enhance the natural bone structure without lengthening the chin and dragging down the face. Oval faces should avoid blunt fringes and harsh crops.

CHOOSE CAREFULLY

Choose your hairdresser carefully. High-street haircuts can be quite limiting because many chains have specific styles for each season and diversification is discouraged. Make sure your hairdresser is working to make you look your best.

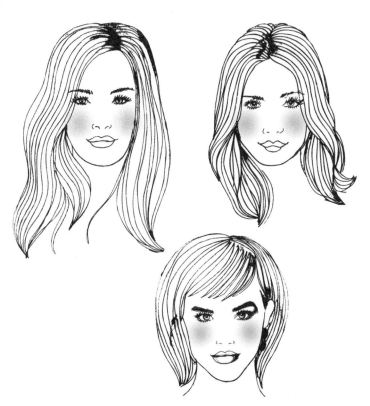

HEART YOUR FRINGE

Heart-shaped faces are perfect for fringes – it will slim down the forehead and accentuate the bones of the lower face. Height on top of the head also works, but beware of long, straight hair or centre partings that can drag the face down.

GO SHORTER

Ageing skin and faces ordinarily look better with lighter, shorter haircuts. This is because long hair can 'drag' the face down, making wrinkles appear worse. Also, the shorter your haircut, the more volume it will appear to have.

HEALTHY HAIR

SLEEP ON SATIN

Sleeping on a silk pillow can help hair stay smooth overnight because the shaft doesn't stick to it as it does to cotton, leaving it smooth and silky come morning. Wrap a silk scarf around your hotel pillow to keep your holiday hair blooming.

DO THE TWIST AND SNIP

One temporary method for removing split ends, though not a solution, is to twist a small strand of hair gently until the damaged and split ends appear, sticking out. Holding a pair of scissors vertically, carefully snip off these ends. You will only be trimming the split ends, not the length.

THICKEN HAIR WITH MASSAGE

One of the signs of ageing is thinning hair. We all lose between 50–100 strands of hair every day but if you're losing more, get a head massage – it will stimulate the roots and help hair growth.

DETOX DULL HAIR

Use a clarifying shampoo once a week to remove build-up of styling products and accumulated conditioner. Product residue weighs down hair, makes it difficult to style and dulls colour.

SCOFF SALMON FOR SHINY TRESSES

Salmon is the number one food for shiny, glossy hair. The fish oils it contains plump up the cuticle and keep hair moisturized without being greasy. Other oily fish are good, too – try sardines, anchovies and mackerel.

KELP IT THICK

Sea kelp supplements are thought to help thicken hair with their marine ingredients, which not only promote hair growth and prevent sun and pollution damage, but also add essential micronutrients to the hair root.

TIE ON A TURBAN

Instead of rubbing hair with a towel, pat it dry instead – wet hair is extremely fragile and rubbing can cause damage to hair shafts. The best way is to wrap hair loosely in a dry towel directly after shampooing to allow the cotton towel to naturally absorb the water. Do not put it on top of the head, which can stretch and knot hair strands, but wrap it along the length, just as it is done in the hair salon.

DETANGLE FROM THE BOTTOM UP

Trying to detangle knots in the hair from the roots down only results in tearing and stretching of the hair shaft. Instead, start at the bottom and work your way slowly up towards the roots, using a leave-in conditioner to help with difficult areas.

HAIR MASKS

LEAVE IN A HONEY SHINE

For a leave-in treatment that gives extra shine, dissolve a teaspoon of honey into 500 ml (1 pint) of warm water. After shampooing, pour the mixture through the hair, distributing evenly. Do not rinse out, and dry as normal.

LIGHTEN UP WITH LEMON

Lemon juice and vinegar are both excellent for oily hair. They will also give lustre to blonde hair and bring out highlights. Never pour vinegar or lemon juice directly onto your hair; dilute them first with water and distribute evenly.

COCONUT SHINE

Coconut has long been known for its moisturizing effects. Make your own hair treat by combining coconut oil with a teaspoon of honey for a ten-minute boosting mask that will rescue dry or damaged hair. Those with very dry or curly hair may benefit from massaging the coconut oil into the hair and leaving it on overnight as it naturally softens, conditions and relaxes the hair.

GET FRUITY FOR EXTRA SHINE

Control oily build-up and add shine with a fruity hair rinse. Heat a sliced orange, a sliced apple and a small slice of melon with 1 litre (2 pints) of water in a saucepan for ten minutes. Strain and allow to cool, then add 500 ml (1 pint) of cider vinegar. Leave for 24 hours before using to rinse hair.

MOISTURIZE WITH OLIVE OIL

Olive oil is nature's great moisturizer. Give yourself a deep-conditioning hot oil hair wrap by massaging gently warmed olive oil into the hair and scalp, then wrap your head in a warm towel (which has been heated in a tumble dryer briefly) for 10–20 minutes. Follow by shampooing, conditioning and drying as usual.

SHAMPOO & CONDITION

WASH THE ROOTS, NOT THE ENDS

When shampooing, concentrate on the roots, not the ends, of the hair – this will clean the greasiest sebum-producing area without stripping the drier parts. Don't worry about not being clean – the shampoo will cleanse the length of the hair as it rinses out.

BANISH BUILD-UP

One of the major causes of problem hair is product build-up, which can be caused by using too much mousse, gel or spray, and not rinsing thoroughly enough. If necessary, shampoo twice to get really clean and always rinse more than you think you need it.

BE PREPARED

If you have a big event to prepare for and you're going to be short of time, or your hair will require styling, wash it the night before and it will be more manageable when you come to style it the next day.

WET IT DOWN

Make sure your hair is completely soaking wet before shampooing. Leave it under the shower for at least a full minute. You will need less shampoo and washing will be much easier.

CUT DOWN ON SHAMPOO

For the shiniest hair you've ever had, halve the amount of shampoo you use (a dessertspoon full should be enough for all but the longest hair) and double the amount of time you spend rinsing.

DEEP CONDITION

If your hair is bleached, give yourself a deep-conditioning treatment once a week to preserve as much moisture as possible in the dehydrated hair shaft and prevent bleach damage spreading through the hair.

SHINE UP WITH BEER

To give hair a really shiny finish and greater manageability, hairdressers recommend rinsing it in beer, which imparts a luscious, rich shine to the hair follicle. Rinse through with water afterwards to avoid smelling like a brewery!

COCONUT CONDITION

Massage hair and scalp with coconut oil to lock moisture into the hair shaft and replenish lost lustre with its light, invisible coating. Coconut also helps to protect against sun and heat damage.

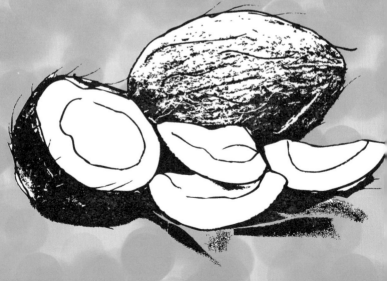

STYLING

BLOW-DRY LIKE A PRO

For super-sleek hair, use a round radial brush and blow-dryer on damp hair. Comb through a serum or thermal protector, then divide your hair into small, 5 cm (2 in) sections. Work section by section from the nape of the neck to the crown. Place the brush underneath the hair and, directing the nozzle of the hairdryer from the roots to the ends, dry along the length. Move the hairdryer constantly. Be careful not to wrap a big section of hair around the brush, otherwise you could get into a tangly mess. Finish each section with a blast of cold air.

SELECT SILICONE

A drop of silicone serum will temporarily coat and smooth the hair cuticle and add shine if your hair is frizzy, dry or damaged. Use only a tiny amount to prevent any build-up and concentrate it on the ends if you have fine or greasy hair.

STAY SMOOTH AND DRY

To dry hair super-straight, use a straightening cream or serum on damp hair. Work down the hair shaft using a hairdryer with a nozzle. If your hair is prone to frizziness, don't dry it upside down or point the airflow upwards, which can roughen up the cuticle – instead, point it down the hair shaft from roots to ends.

FORESTALL THE FRIZZ

If you suffer from frizzy hair, dry hair completely before leaving the house. Kinking or frizzing can occur if hair is even just a tiny bit damp when you go out in the wind and air.

FIGHT THE FRIZZ

If your hair is curly or very prone to frizz, especially in damp weather, try to use a wide-toothed comb, which separates the hairs, rather than a brush. Avoid handling the hair too much and apply serum or a leave-in conditioner with the fingers, smoothing the hair into manageable locks or large ringlets.

FRENCH PLAIT

For a great way to create waves, especially on thick hair, get a friend to give you a French plait while hair is still damp, then leave it in for several hours and use fingers to tease out the curls.

STOP THE STATIC

To remedy flyaway, static hair, which is especially a problem in hot, dry weather, spray hairspray on your brush and brush through your hair. Alternatively spritz with water. Always use a moisturizing shampoo.

START AT THE BACK

Apply styling products first to the back of the hair, where you have most hair, working your way forwards to the front sections. This will ensure even distribution and prevent you from adding too much product to the top of the head.

DON'T HEAT EXTENSIONS

If you want to style or curl acrylic hair extensions, be sure to use rollers with no thermal styling products and take care using hot blow-dryers or other styling tools. Most extensions are not made of real hair and may burn. To prolong the life of your extensions, whether they are natural or acrylic, never sleep with wet hair and do not try to dye them yourself at home – always visit a salon for colour.

DRY NATURALLY

Allow hair to dry naturally as often as possible to restore hair health, rather than always reaching for the hairdryer and styling tools. If you hate your frizzy curls, apply a serum and twist large ringlets around your fingers as your hair air-dries – this creates large sleek curls rather than frizzy ones and you may love your new look.

GET SILKY SHINE

Smooth silk can boost the natural shine of your hair and help smooth down follicles. Wrap a silk scarf around your hairbrush and 'brush' your hair with it to add lustrous shine.

TRY TOUSLED TRESSES

Instead of leaving hair looking groomed to within an inch of its life, try spraying a mist of volumizing lotion onto it and style with fingers only to add texture and avoid that over-brushed look.

CHOOSE VELCRO FOR FINE HAIR

Velcro rollers provide soft curl and full body, and can be used on either damp or dry hair. They are good choices for short or fine hair and hair that breaks easily, since they don't need to be clipped in place.

NEW DAY, NEW LOOK

For a new look without a cut, simply change your parting. If you are used to a side parting, a centre one can really make your features stand out and give you a fresher, younger look.

GO LOOSE FOR ROLLERS

Never wind rollers too tightly, or you could end up with hair loss and damage as the hair is stretched, torn or pulled out from the root. Remember, hair contracts when drying, so if you're putting them on wet hair, give yourself a bit of extra room.

STYLING TOOLS

DON'T NEGLECT BRUSHES

Just like your hair, your brushes, combs and styling tools need regular washing to maintain tiptop form. Use shampoo or mild detergent to keep them sparkling clean.

DON'T BE CAUGHT WITHOUT A PADDLE

With their large, flat bases, paddle brushes are great for smoothing out medium-length to long hair. If you want to blow-dry your tresses straight and shiny, hold the brush perpendicular to the hair and aim the blow-dryer at the base of the brush.

DON'T KEEP DAMAGED GOODS

When the bristles of your hairbrush start looking damaged, bent or frayed, or the brush starts losing bristles, it's time to replace your hairbrush. Over-used bristles can damage and pull hair, causing split ends and tearing.

BUY THE BEST BRISTLES

Avoid hairbrushes with synthetic bristles, which can be harsh on both the hair and the skin of the scalp. Opt for combs or natural fibres instead, such as boar bristles. If you can only afford synthetic varieties, choose ones with round-tipped or ball ends.

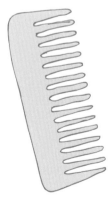

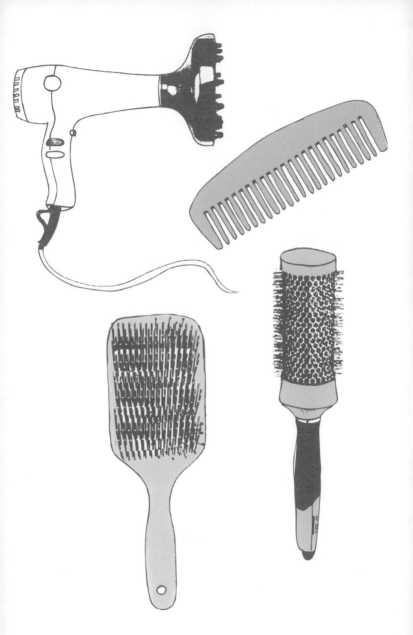

BODY BEAUTIFUL

BODY MASKS

LOSE INCHES WITH CLAY

Clay products are great home spa choices for inch loss because they leach excess fluids out of the skin and help tone and tighten skin, especially if used with compressing bandages to squish cells together. The more absorbent the clay, the more inches will be lost.

REVITALIZE WITH ROSE

Make a revitalizing body mask with rose and lime by mixing rosewater and lime juice with a little glycerine and use the lotion on dry skin after a bath. Store in the fridge if you want to keep it for more than a few days.

PLAY DEAD

Dead sea salts are fantastic for replenishing skin health and boosting circulation. For best results, lie back in a bath and gently massage skin to absorb the salty goodness.

MAKE YOUR OWN WRAP

The simplest wrap is clay with added salt, which is highly absorbent. Warm some water, add ingredients then dip in bandages and wrap yourself in them. You can add herbs such as rose petals, camomile or ginger powder, if required.

BOOST CIRCULATION

If you're using a body mask, tighten up problem areas using gently wrapped plastic wrap or bandages, which can improve circulation by tightening the skin and helping it to release toxins.

HOT AND COLD

Bath temperatures can be used therapeutically, but may not achieve the relaxing treat you are looking for. Cold baths reduce swelling by constricting blood vessels while hot ones relieve muscle soreness and eliminate body toxins.

DRINK BE WARM

Choose a warm room for body masks and treatments so the mixture stays warm for longer and doesn't dry out. Warmer surroundings boost your circulation, which brings more blood to the surface and helps the mask do its work.

MAXIMIZE THE MASK

To maximize the effects of a detoxifying body mask, take a cool or lukewarm bath afterwards and then, two or three days later, take a hot bath which will open up the pores and release any accumulated toxins from the skin.

CELLULITE-BUSTERS

UNDERSTAND ENDERMOLOGIE

Endermologie is a salon-based deep-tissue suction treatment that rolls and pinches fatty tissues to break down subcutaneous fat deposits, toxins and retained water. After a number of sessions, you should notice improvements in the overall texture and appearance of the skin.

DRY BRUSH DIMPLED SKIN

A favourite three-pronged method for dealing with cellulite is to first eliminate toxins from your diet, such as alcohol, caffeine and processed food, then to break it down by using dry skin brushing and lymphatic drainage massage and, finally, to firm up the skin with a good anti-cellulite tightening serum or body cream.

GO TO GROUNDS

To reduce cellulite, cut out coffee from your diet, but don't throw the grounds away – instead, use them damp as a super-stimulating rub for areas prone to cellulite, working towards the heart in big strokes.

MASSAGE IN DEEPLY

Always massage in a cellulite cream, working from the extremities toward the heart and in circular motions – it's the massaging effect that's as beneficial as the cream.

FRAGRANCE

VIAL IT IN YOUR BAG

Invest in a small vial and decant some from the bottle if you want to carry scent around with you in your handbag, or choose a small travel size. If you take the whole bottle with you, and expose it to light or heat, the scent may go off prematurely.

THROUGH THE WOODS

Chypre scents are based on mossy and fern notes that are often combined with jasmine, rose or citrus, and are ideal if you like warm, aromatic scents.

KEEP IT BOXED UP

Keeping perfumes in their boxes shields them from light, which can cause chemical changes in their make-up and helps them last longer than if exposed to light.

GET SCENTS-IBLE

Perfume and scent can change the way you feel. To give yourself a lift, opt for citrus scents or vanilla, and for sexy evenings, try musk or rose.

GET IN A DIFFERENT MOOD

Because most eau de toilettes are potent for only four to five hours, you can change fragrances throughout the day to suit your mood. Not many people have a 'signature' scent they stick to for all occasions.

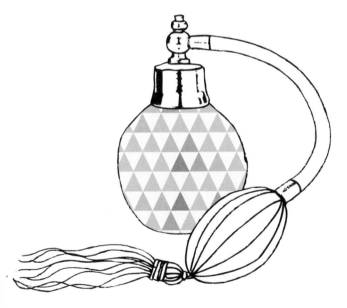

DON'T SPRAY ONTO SILK

While it is great to have your fragrance on your clothes and hair, avoid spraying directly onto fabric. Many materials, especially silk, will stain permanently.

LIGHT OR HEAVY?

Choose your type of scent according to how you will wear it – eau fraîche only lasts for an hour or two; with eau de toilettes 20 per cent of the scent will last all day; with eau de parfum 30 per cent lasts all day; and with perfume 50 per cent lasts all day.

ORIENTAL FRAGRANCES

Spicy musks, woods and ambers form the basis of this sultry and seductive family of fragrances. They are heavier and longer lasting, making them popular for evening.

WEAR IT NAKED

Don't simply add perfume on your way out the door – it needs the warmth of your skin to interact with the oils. Scent should be worn directly on your skin under your clothes for lasting effect. Put it on pulse points low on the body as it will rise with your body heat. Be like Marilyn Monroe and only wear Chanel No. 5 to bed!

A NOSE FOR NEW SCENTS

When trying out a new scent, wait up to five hours for it to develop on your skin – this way you will first smell the top notes, then the middle at about two to four hours later (the important notes) and finally the full base note.

HAIR REMOVAL

WARM UP INGROWING HAIRS

For ingrown pubic hairs along the bikini line, hold a hot
compress against ingrown spots for ten minutes a couple of times
a day to soften the skin and help the hairs work their way out.

CALM DOWN WITH CAMOMILE

Many spas use camomile wax, which is normal wax infused with
calming camomile, which can ease pain and redness following
waxing. If you have sensitive skin, this can mean happier hair
removal – ask your beautician for advice.

EXFOLIATE BEFORE YOU WAX

To avoid ingrown hairs post-waxing, remove dead skin cells,
which might obstruct the hair beforehand by exfoliating the area
to be waxed. Because skin will be softer, you are less likely to
develop ingrown hairs.

BLEACH AWAY DOWN

If you have downy hair on your forehead or in front of your ears,
rub a freshly cut lemon over the hair and leave for five to ten
minutes before rinsing off for a natural bleaching agent which
won't make them bright white.

WAIT AND SEE

If you have ingrown pubic hairs, don't be tempted to over-
exfoliate as this could cause further skin trauma, which may
result in sore spots, infections or more serious irritation of the
skin. Wait until it's gone and then exfoliate.

SHAKE AND WAX

When waxing your hair at home, first shake talcum powder over the area to be waxed as this helps the strip to rip and be more effective.

POP A PILL

If you find the pain of waxing or epilating too much to bear, lessen the pain by taking paracetamol or ibuprofen 15 minutes beforehand to help reduce your suffering.

CONDITION AND SHAVE

If you have run out of shaving foam, use hair conditioner when shaving legs. Because it's smooth, it will stop the skin dragging and help you shave smoothly without stretching the skin.

WET SHAVE FOR SMOOTH SKIN

As any barber will tell you, wet shaves are the most effective. Before shaving, wet the hair as well as the skin, use a foam or mousse specifically for shaving, and pull the skin taut to ensure a smooth finish. Work upwards with long, even strokes.

AVOID THE TIME OF THE MONTH

In the few days before your period, when hormone levels in the body are out of balance, waxing can be more painful then at other times of the month, so check your diary before you de-fuzz.

KEEP YOUR COOL

Avoid saunas, hot baths, exercise or sunbathing for 24 hours after waxing. All of these can raise your body temperature, which means you may sweat more, causing irritation to treated areas.

HANDS & FEET

TAKE OUT TOBACCO STAINS

Rub tobacco-stained fingers and nails with half a freshly cut lemon for five to ten minutes to help bleach skin naturally without drying it out. Rubbing the back of the hands with lemon will also fade age spots.

SUN-PROTECT YOUR HANDS

In summer, add a layer of sunscreen to your hands or use a hand cream with SPF to protect skin against dryness, wrinkles and premature ageing.

SCRUB WELL

Mix a paste of almond oil and salt in the palm of one hand and use to scrub the back of your hands and over your knuckles – your hands will feel and look silky smooth.

BOWL HANDS OVER

For hands that are smooth and wrinkle free, soak them in a bowl of warm water for five minutes before drying and applying your favourite hand cream. The water soaks into the skin and the cream forms a barrier, locking it in and easing aches and pains at the same time.

GET SOME WRIST ACTION

To ease tired hands and give yourself a circulation boost, hold both hands in front of you with palms facing inwards, loosen their wrist grip and flap them backwards and forwards. Feel them tingle as the blood rushes to them.

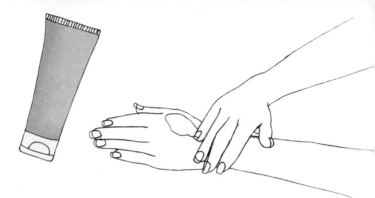

KEEP HANDS YOUNG

Take care of your hands before they give away your secrets.
Hand skin is frequently neglected, but it's often the real telltale
sign of age. Invest in a rich hand cream day and night to keep
your hands looking young and tender.

BAN WARTS WITH DANDELION

Dandelion stems have long been believed to help banish warts.
Apply the juice of a dandelion stem two or three times daily for
several weeks.

BE A BAREFOOT BEAUTY

Allow feet to breathe and you'll avoid many unsightly problems
like fungal infections. Use natural, breathable fibres whenever
possible for socks and try to go barefoot for at least an hour a day.

SEE YOUR PODIATRIST

If you're suffering corns or callouses, see a podiatrist, also called
a chiropodist, who is skilled in dealing with all kinds of foot
problems, from verrucas to deformities, and will do more than a
pedicurist to help you solve these problems. They will also assess
how you walk and the shape of your foot to see if there are any
physical reasons for the cause of your problems, and be able to
advise and provide surgery for persistent ingrown nails.

SOCK IT TO DRY FEET

Before bed, exfoliate feet and rub in cream or oil, then pull on a pair of socks to help them make the most of their newfound moisture all night long. When you wake up, they'll be as soft as a baby's!

TREAT ATHLETE'S FOOT WITH TEA TREE

Tea tree oil, with its naturally astringent and antibacterial properties, can help prevent the spread of athlete's foot by drying out skin and making it hard for the fungus to spread.

PUMICE AWAY HARD SKIN

To remove hard skin on feet, rub with a pumice after soaking the feet for at least ten minutes to soften problem areas, such as the balls of the feet and the heels. The natural stone will not only remove dead skin but will boost circulation to the area, encouraging regeneration.

DON'T RAZOR IT OFF

Never remove hard skin with a razor blade, or allow nail technicians or pedicurists to use one on you. This will only spur the skin into producing harder skin to replace it, which defeats the purpose of having it removed. Your therapist may use a strong exfoliator scrub or solution to aid in the removal of tough skin.

HOME SPA

SOME LIKE IT NOT HOT

For a relaxing bath, make sure the water is pleasantly warm rather than hot, which can stimulate your system and cause the skin to slacken and dehydrate as a result. Always test the water before you enter.

COMPRESS STRESS

Make a quick stress-relieving compress by adding a few drops of lavender or camomile essential oil to a bowl of warm water and soaking a cotton cloth in it for five minutes, then applying to face and neck as a compress and breathing deeply. Repeat three times.

GET A GOMMAGE

For a home spa gommage (salt glow) as good as any salon, mix ground sea salt with 12 drops of a stimulating essential oil such as grapefruit, lemon or thyme. Make a paste by adding enough water to spread easily and apply in brisk circular strokes, especially on hips and thighs.

COPY CLEOPATRA

Cleopatra was famous for her smooth skin and milk baths. Follow her beauty secret by adding 3 cups of powdered milk or fresh milk to a warm bath. The lactic acid in the milk will soften and gently exfoliate skin.

GARDEN HERB SOAK

Place a bunch of garden herbs such as rose, lavender and rosemary in a tea strainer and hang it from the running tap in your bath for a healing soak from your own botanical garden!

TRY CRYOTHERAPY

Steal a salon secret (cyrotherapy is extreme cold applied for therapeutic purposes) for your own home – after applying a face-firming treatment, place an ice cube inside a small plastic bag and gently rub over the face and eye area for several minutes to plump up and tone the skin.

BOOST BATHING WITH EPSOM

When Epsom salts (aka magnesium sulphate) are absorbed through the skin in a bath, they help to draw toxins from the body, reduce swelling and relax muscles as the skin cools afterwards. Mix a handful of Epsom salts with a handful of sea salt and a splash of bath oil or olive oil.

SCENT-SATIONAL PLEASURE

An essential oil diffuser will add to the overall effect of the at-home spa experience. Choose either a relaxing oil such as lavender or an invigorating one like rosemary, according to your mood. Play a CD of nature sounds, turn off all phones and retreat from the world for a few hours.

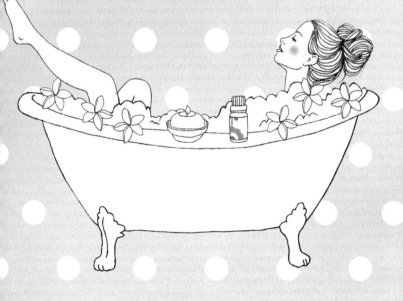

LUSCIOUS LEGS

SPARKLE AT SOIREES

Don't limit make-up to your face and décolletage. Add some glamorous sparkle to your arms and legs for a sexy evening look. Add a little gold highlighter to your moisturizer and smooth down shins and across shoulder and collarbones to give them shape and shimmer.

GO CITRUS FOR VARICOSE VEINS

To reduce the appearance of varicose veins, add extra citrus fruits, grapes, cherries and apricots to your diet. If eaten regularly, these foods can help improve the elasticity of blood vessels.

GO ROUND IN CIRCLES

Always apply your moisturizer or body scrub in a circular motion from the ankle up as this boosts the circulation of the blood in the legs, facilitating lymphatic drainage and boosting circulation and, therefore, skin health.

BOOST CIRCULATION

Sometimes, 'big looking' legs may not be fat, but appear heavy because of bad circulation. Put your legs and feet up above hip level for half an hour a day to help fluid flow. If you suffer from varicose veins, this will also help reduce the strain on blood vessels.

JET LEGS WITH COLD WATER

Finish your shower with a jet of cold water aimed at your lower legs. Not only will this stimulate skin, but it will help constrict the blood vessels in the area, too, boosting the overall appearance.

MASSAGE

KNEAD BETWEEN THE LINES

Reduce forehead lines caused by tension by using a soft, shallow pinch to relax muscles. Make your hand into a fist, then pinch skin between your thumb and index finger for gentle stimulation.

BE A TENNIS PRO

Instead of shelling out for an expensive salon massage, make your own back relaxer by lying on your back on a couple of used tennis balls, positioned at the top of your buttocks or your lower back with your knees pointing up and your feet flat on the floor. Then roll around to release tension in the back area.

GET YOUR HAND IN

Give yourself a circulation mini-boost when applying hand cream by using small, circular movements to rub the cream into your knuckles and joints. Use your thumbs to massage the backs of your hands.

BREAST UPLIFT

The thin skin on your breasts is prone to sagging and toxin build-up. Massage problems away using almond oil and gentle sweeping strokes from the underside up into your armpits.

FINISH WITH A BATH

After your massage, soak in a bath for a ten-minute relaxation. Aromatherapy oils are particularly beneficial at this time because you will already be relaxed and have stimulated skin, which will make the oils more efficient.

NURTURE YOUR NECK

With your right hand, gently massage the left side of your neck at the shoulder in a rhythmic motion, working from the base to the ear, and moving slightly round to the back as you do so, in circular strokes. Repeat on the right side of the neck using your left hand. Finish with the fingers of both hands working the back of your neck.

TAKE THE PINCH

Stimulate circulation in your facial skin by pinching the jawline. Start at the chin, pinching with your thumbs underneath and your fingers on top, and holding for ten seconds. Move along the lower jawbone until you reach the earlobes. Aim for four to five pinches to cover the area.

NAILS

MAXIMIZE NAIL GROWTH

To stimulate nail growth, massage the base of the nails with cuticle oil several times a day. This will stimulate and nourish the nail bed, encouraging new growth.

HEAT UP YOUR NAILS

Bend the fingers of the hands in towards the palms and rub the nails for a minute to give your nails a boost of oxygen and nutrient-rich blood, which will reduce nail problems.

CHILL OUT

Nail varnish will stay fresher for longer if it's kept in the refrigerator, which will help prevent it separating and clogging due to heat and light damage.

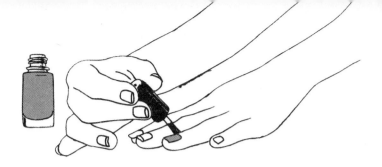

EXTEND YOUR RANGE

If you have difficulty growing all your nails to the same length, fake it with extensions. Gel versions are glued onto the real nail, then cut and shaped. These are less irritating than acrylic versions, which are longer lasting and stronger but more difficult to remove.

BASE, COLOUR AND TOP

Always follow the three-step programme to varnish your nails: first apply a base coat to protect the nail from discolouring, then apply two coats of the colour, and finish with a clear, glossy top coat for extra shine and to guard against chips.

GO SOFT, NOT LOOSE

The excessive use of nail hardeners that contain formaldehyde can cause lots of nail problems, including peeling, splitting and loose nails, when the nail plate separates from the nail bed. If you suspect this is the source of your problems, go easy on products and use a perfume-free nail cream.

PRIME NAILS WITH PROTEIN

When nails easily crack or break they can be a permanent worry. Weak nails may be caused by a protein deficiency in the diet. Increase nutritional intake by eating more lean meat, fish, fresh fruit and vegetables and use a nail cream to help hydrate.

DO THE DIP TIP

To speed up nail varnish drying, run nails under cold water for ten minutes to help the varnish form a hard, knock-free coating in no time at all.

BREAK FREE OF BRITTLE NAILS

Brittle nails can be caused by over-exposure to the sun, a poor diet or the prolonged use of commercial nail hardeners. Avoid the use of hardeners or varnishes containing formaldehyde, which has a drying effect on nails.

LET YOUR NAILS BREATHE

Leave nails unpainted for at least a few days a month to help them breathe. This will reduce yellowing and staining from polish on the nail and give it a chance to recover health and glow.

CARE FOR CUTICLES

Massage a cuticle oil or cream into the base of the nails at least once a day to prevent dryness, scarring and hangnails. If cuticles are damaged and painful, gently apply a moisturizer twice daily until they heal.

TWINKLE THOSE TOES

Pale, subtle varnishes are wasted on summer toenails – open-toed sandals cry out for bright colours, such as shocking pink, or sparkly and metallic hues.

CLING ON

Wait at least 45 minutes after painting your toenails before putting on closed-toe shoes, but if you absolutely must go out, wrap your toes in plastic wrap before slipping on shoes to avoid smudges.

BE A SQUARE

Clip and file toenails squarely in line with the ends of the toes so that the growth does not push into the surrounding tissue, which can be ugly and painful.

FILE WITHOUT FRICTION

When filing nails, work in one direction from the outside edge toward the centre, rather than sawing back and forth, as too much friction can cause splits and tears. Angle the file slightly so you are filing away more from underneath the nail than on top. Avoid metal emery boards, which can be too harsh for nail ends.

LET SPOTS GROW OUT

White spots on nails are usually the result of trauma to the nail or nail bed. Give the spots time to grow out and make an effort to be gentle when manicuring your nails – prodding beneath the cuticles, where new growth is generated, can cause white spots and damaged nails.

BACK TO BASES

If you have yellow nails, it could be because you haven't used a base coat underneath your regular nail colour. Yellow patches or streaks that don't go away could be due to fungal infections that might need treatment.

HARD AS NAILS

For weak or brittle nails, apply a nail strengthener every day for a week, then remove and leave the nails to rest for a few days before repeating for another week, if necessary. Make sure you file the nails into a square shape rather than an oval, which will avoid weakening the sides and causing splits and tears.

ZAP FLECKS WITH ZINC

White flecks in the nails are caused by injury or, in some cases, a deficiency of zinc. Supplement your diet with eggs, shellfish, chickpeas and lentils, all good sources of dietary zinc.

COLOUR THAT LASTS

Colour wears off the tips of polished nails first. To make your manicure last longer, take the colour over the edge of the nail to underneath – the added polish will protect against chipping.

SALON SECRETS

BRAVE MICRODERMABRASION

This skin-booster uses aluminium oxide particles to slough off the outermost layers, leaving complexions brighter and evening out tone and colour. There are home-based alternatives, but professional is best to reduce redness and irritation post-treatment.

LASER YOUR VEINS

The treatment works by using lasers to create heat in the veins, which damages the lining of the blood vessel and causes the walls of the vessel to stick together and seal themselves off. The vein is gradually absorbed by the body and disappear.

DIP INTO THE DEAD SEA

You can buy these products for use at home, but the more powerful ingredients are reserved for salon formulations. The treatments use the mineral-rich mud from the Dead Sea to detoxify and revitalize skin.

PEEL AWAY PROBLEMS

Facial chemical peels should always be performed by a trained therapist or dermatologist, as the concentrations of skin-clearing chemicals are higher than in home-based treatments, which means they penetrate more deeply and have more radical results.

DON'T BE FAZED BY LASERS

Lasers are now being used in salons to resurface, smooth and lighten skin and to even out pigmentation, age marks and acne scars. Because lasers can inflict damage, you should always visit a professional to have them administered.

QUICK-TIME MAKEOVERS

If you are time-poor and need a quick makeover for a special event, book an express treatment. Many hair and beauty salons offer a cut and colour combined with body treatments, such as manicures, massages and brow shaping.

FILL IT WITH FILLERS

To fill out acne scars, frown lines and wrinkles, dermal fillers are popular for the areas Botox doesn't reach – such as the laugh lines and for pumping up thin lips. Choose a biodegradable hyaluronic acid-based filler rather than a permanent one – the results last less time but there is less chance of unsightly lumps and movement.

PULSE AWAY PIGMENT

Pulsed light technology is an alternative to lasers. With this salon treatment, pulses of intense, concentrated light are directed onto the skin and absorbed by the melanin in pigmented lesions, such as age, sun and liver spots, which evens out pigmentation. The technique is also used for hair removal and blemishes.

LIGHT UP YOUR LIFE

New salon treatments that involve an application of yellow light to reduce the bacterial count in skin can reduce acne by up to half after just one treatment. Called Light Therapy, it's a miracle for problem skin.

THERMO-TARGET THREAD VEINS

Thermo-coagulation is a vein-removal technique based on a high-frequency wave producing a thermal lesion that reduces the vein. A very fine needle is inserted into the vein and it disappears instantaneously.

HANDLE HYLAFORM WITH CARE

Dermal injections involve plumping up facial lines and wrinkles by injecting small amounts of the filler into them. Hylaform uses hyaluronic acid, from rooster combs, as its key compound, which could cause allergic reactions. Non-animal derived hyaluronic is used in Restylane and Perlane.

OPT FOR SCLEROTHERAPY

Sclerotherapy removes thread veins from the legs by injecting a special solution into the vein via an ultra-fine needle. The sides of the vein stick together and the vein eventually fades away. The smaller the vein, the easier it is to treat. It may also remedy such symptoms as aching, burning, swelling and cramps.

MASSAGE AWAY PUFFINESS

A great instant pick-me-up if you are suffering from puffy or problem skin is a manual lymphatic drainage (MLD) massage, which boosts circulation, detoxifies and reduces fluid build-up. It is used to improve cellulite and stretch marks, too.

NATURAL BEAUTY

SMOOTH & FIRM

LOOK LEAN BY GOING GREEN
Did you know that green tea can help you lose weight by
stimulating your basal metabolic rate to help you burn calories
more easily? Two cups a day is ample.

BE COOL
Hot showers can sting skin and cause moisture loss. Instead,
finish off hot days with a lukewarm or tepid shower blast.

FIRM WITH A GEL
The delicate skin on the neck and upper chest is a target for sun
damage and ages fast. In fact, you may notice the neck lines and
crevices before you notice them on your face. The best formulas
for this area are gel- or serum-based and not only deliver a
sunscreen and anti-ageing moisturizer, but fade age spots and
firm loose skin, albeit temporarily.

GRAB A GRAPEFRUIT
Grapefruit is an excellent choice for a healthy fruit that will
make you look good. It is a natural diuretic, which prevents
bloating and water retention, and helps you stay slim. Choose
it as a healthy starter or a mid-afternoon snack. Many beauty
products contain grapefruit purely for its reinvigorating scent.

MASSAGE AS YOU MOISTURIZE

When you apply a body oil or lotion, do so using massage techniques: use sweeping, upward motions towards your heart to give your lymphatic drainage a boost. Taking time to really work the oil into your skin will help it penetrate and imbue a lustrous glow.

GIVE YOURSELF THE BRUSH-OFF

Improving skin circulation – by body brushing, scrubbing and massage – will even out skin tone and boost oxygenation of the cells, leading to fresher, smoother, glowing skin all year round.

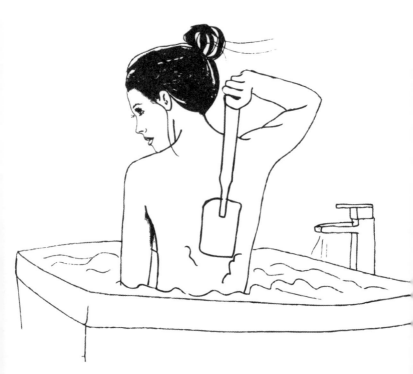

SUN WORSHIP

HEAD FOR A SCREEN TEST
Don't be tempted to use intensive moisturizers or conditioners in your hair in the hope that they'll keep your locks protected in the sun – the sun burns them up, which can make hair even drier. Instead, use a hair-specific sunscreen for ultimate protection.

BE A SHADY LADY
Take care of the delicate skin around the eyes with a pair of polarized sunglasses. Wraparound styles that fully cover the whole eye area and the sides of the face are best, as they protect the skin prone to crows' feet and fine under-eye lines.

KEEP CREAM COOL
Sun cream is more effective when it's kept cool, so make sure you leave it in the shade if you're on the beach, or the sun's heat could denature the active ingredients and make it less effective.

BE A CITY SLICKER
Skin isn't only exposed to the sun on the beach in summer – in town choose a tinted moisturizer with built-in sunscreen to give you a healthy glow without the damage.

DO THE DOSE RIGHT
For a sunscreen to live up to its SPF rating, 2 mg should be applied for every square centimetre (⅛ inch) of exposed skin, which means on average you should be using 100 mg for every four whole-body applications. Most people don't use anything like enough.

DON'T BE HASTY

When you moisturize before applying a sunscreen, make sure you leave 15–30 minutes for the moisturizer to soak into the skin first. This will ensure that the sunblock works correctly.

KEEP HAIR SMOOTH

UV rays, chlorine and salt can damage and dry hair, so protect hair as well as skin in the sun using a sunscreen spray, mask or cream specially formulated for the hair. These products will lock moisture in and reduce colour fade.

TAN WITH TANGERINES

Antioxidant vitamins A, C and E – found in red, yellow and orange fruit and vegetables – can help limit damage to skin from the sun's rays by mopping up damaging free radicals in the body.

PROTECT YOUR FACE

The skin on your face and neck is among the thinnest and most sensitive on your body. To prevent damage from the sun's rays, cover up with a wide-brimmed hat, especially in the danger hours from 11 am to 3 pm. This will also protect your hair from looking sun-frazzled.

PUCKER UP

Don't forget lips need sun protection too – the skin on them is thinner than anywhere else on your face, and overexposure to the sun and elements can leave them dry and coarse. Use a sunscreen specially formulated for the lips with a minimum of SPF 15.

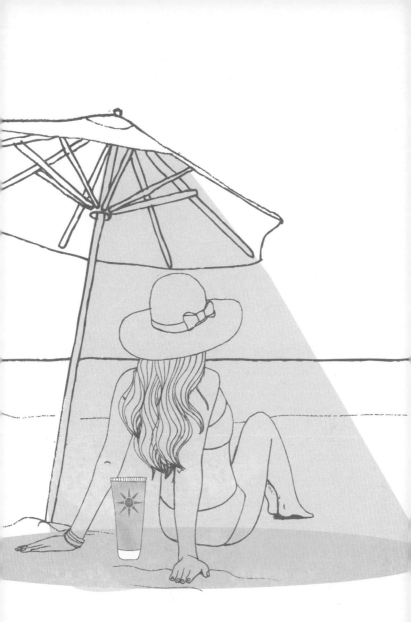

SUNLESS TANNING

DO YOUR PREP

Self-tanners contain a chemical called DHA (dihydroxyacetone), a colourless sugar that stains the uppermost layer of skin, so it's better to get the application right in the first place than try to correct mistakes. Try the 3-step rule: exfoliate, moisturize, apply.

DRY SKIN MAY GO DARK

Dry skin around knees, elbows and ankles picks up self-tan colour more, leading to dark patches. Instead of applying tan neat, mix it with moisturizer for these areas.

EXFOLIATE DAILY

Prepare your skin for self-tanning by exfoliating daily for the three or four days before you apply it and using moisturizer liberally following exfoliation to build up smoothness and hydration in the skin and prevent uneven streaks.

HAVE A CLOSE SHAVE

Shaving not only removes hairs, it also serves to exfoliate the skin by stretching off the top layer, so it's a great choice the day before you apply self-tan. But avoid shaving for a day or two afterwards as it could weaken the tan.

MOISTURIZE MODERATELY

Too much moisturizer is one of the biggest fake tan mistakes – it creates a barrier between the skin and the tan, making the tanning dye less effective and more prone to slipping and streaks. Wait until the body cream has soaked in before applying fake tan.

HANDS OFF THE TAN!

Prevent tell-tale orange palms by applying a tiny amount of silicone-based 'frizz-control' hair product to your palms, which blocks the pigment from absorbing into your skin.

INNER BEAUTY

COUNT YOUR UNITS

Alcohol causes changes in the body's circulation system, which can lead to broken veins on cheeks and nose. Keep your intake down to a maximum of 14 units a week and try to have at least one completely dry day.

POLISH WITH PORRIDGE

For a morning glow, breakfast on porridge with skimmed milk, topped with flaxseeds and blueberries and a glass of orange juice, – all the best ingredients for healthy skin.

SCOFF FRUIT FOR HEALTHY SKIN

Fruit is essential for healthy skin, not only because of all the vitamins and minerals, but also because it contains high levels of water, which also serve to keep skin hydrated. Pimples or congested skin in the forehead area is often a sign of constipation or blockage in the lymphatic systems, which can be relieved by eating plenty of fruit and vegetables.

GO FOR GRAPEFRUIT

Eat well for gorgeous-looking skin, by fixing yourself a lunch of grilled shrimp salad with grapefruit and watercress. These ingredients contain high levels of zinc and antioxidants to boost skin healing. Top it with parsley, which is rich in vitamin A, chlorophyll, vitamin B12, folic acid, vitamin C and iron – all good for skin health.

NATURAL REMEDIES

ALMOND EYES

Almond oil is a super all-round moisturizer. Use it on your lips and around your mouth, as a hand moisturizer or as a gentle eye make-up remover to smooth away wrinkles.

END ITCHING WITH ALOE

For those suffering extreme dryness or eczema, creams containing high levels of lavender and aloe vera can stop the itching. These ingredients have fast-acting, skin-soothing properties.

CURE SPOTS WITH FENUGREEK

Fenugreek leaves infused in a small amount of water and made into a paste can be used to target pimples, blackheads and dryness if applied and left overnight. Wash off with warm water in the morning.

COME TO THE OIL

Essential oils are relaxing, detoxifying and nourishing. They are absorbed very easily and won't leave your face shiny. Rose oil is particularly noted for its soothing properties and restores suppleness to mature skins – blend a few drops with patchouli and geranium oils in a carrier oil and apply a small amount nightly.

RITES OF MASSAGE

Massage can help uneven skin tone by boosting circulation and encouraging the migration of pigment cells under the skin, which evens out patchiness. It is especially good for circulation danger spots like the chin, jaw and upper arms.

JOJOBA FOR HAIR DRYNESS

Jojoba oil is waxy and rich in antioxidants; it will condition and nourish the hair shaft, leaving hair moisturized, smooth and sleek. Leave on overnight for a deep treatment, shampooing it out in the morning, or look for conditioner that contains it. Although plant-derived, jojoba is closer in make-up to sebum than to traditional vegetable oils.

BOOST SKIN HEALTH WITH APRICOTS

Apricots are a rich source of betacarotene, folic acid and iron, all of which boost skin health and help combat damaging free radicals and toxins from the environment and additives in food and cosmetics. The vitamin A helps keep skin soft and supple, and repairs skin cells and tissues.

BE AN OMEGA-3 BEAUTY

Omega-3 oils, found in high levels in oily fish like mackerel, sardines and salmon, can benefit skin by reducing inflammation and helping the elimination of toxins.

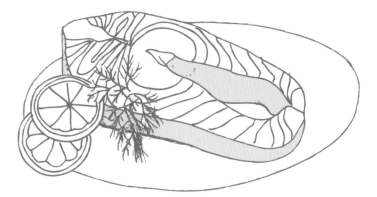

PRESS AWAY PROBLEMS

In acupuncture, the area above your kneecap (measure the
length of your kneecap and move exactly this distance above
it and 2.5 cm (1in) towards your inner thigh) is linked to skin
problems. Press on each leg at the spot for at least a minute to
reduce itching and inflammation of the skin.

GET EVEN WITH PRIMROSE

Many natural cosmetics include evening primrose oil as one
of their key components. The oil has a high concentration of
omega-3 oils and gamma-linolenic acid (GLA) that have been
shown to help prevent and ease symptoms of psoriasis, eczema
and other skin conditions. It also helps maintain the skin's water
barrier. The essential fatty acids keep nails healthy and prevent
cracks, and nourish the scalp and hair.

SEED THE BENEFITS

Pumpkin, sesame and sunflower seeds are packed with skin-
rejuvenating elements like essential fats, vitamins and minerals.
Include them in your diet at least three or four times a week for
best results.

EASE ECZEMA WITH LINOLEIC ACID

Linoleic acid, found in many supplements and most nuts and
seeds, is a powerful omega-6 oil, which helps eczema sufferers
more than olive or fish oils.

SALT OF THE EARTH

Salt baths encourage gentle detoxification of your whole body,
and are particularly good for problem skin and fluid retention.
Taken at the end of the day, they can also reduce tension and
promote a good night's sleep.

TEA TREE WORKS A TREAT

Lavender and tea tree oil, as well as witch hazel, have natural antiseptic properties that can help prevent spots and bites becoming infected. Manuka honey is also a natural antiseptic, though it's a lot stickier!

SLEEP WELL WITH SANDALWOOD

As well as being an excellent moisturizer, a few drops of sandalwood oil in your bath can help decrease tension and relieve insomnia. Traditionally, it is also a natural antidepressant.

END THE DAY WITH LAVENDER

Lavender oil is skin-soothing, can help alleviate aches and pains, and is a marvellous sleep aid. Try adding five or six drops of the essential oil into a warm bath before bed to ensure you get your beauty sleep.

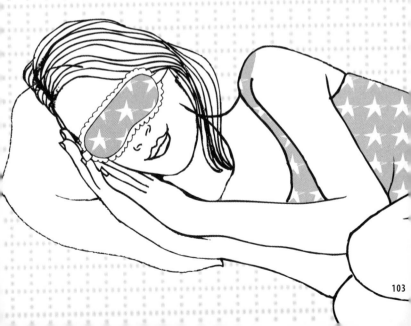

SUPPLEMENTS

AFA FOR HEALTHY HAIR

The supplement AFA (aphanizomenon flos-aquae) is a blue-green algae that contains all eight essential amino acids. It gives shine to hair, stimulates nail health, increases mental and physical alertness, promotes healthy intestinal flora and provides stable blood sugar levels.

GET THE MSM MESSAGE

MSM (methylsulfonylmethane) is a naturally occurring nutrient found in protein-rich eggs, meat and fish. It is often called nature's beauty mineral, as it promotes a clear complexion, glossy hair and fast and effective recovery from injury, including scar healing.

B FREE OF LIVER SPOTS

A supplement high in B vitamins is thought to help clear up liver spots on face and hands, which can be unsightly. You can also find B vitamins in meat, fortified cereals and yeast extract.

HORSE AROUND

Horse chestnut is an age-old remedy for treating varicose veins, haemorrhoids and other problems linked with poor circulation. Take it in tablet form to boost and tone of your circulatory system.

BEAT SPOTS WITH EVENING PRIMROSE

Evening primrose oil, taken as daily capsules, has been shown to help skin stay supple and spot-free as well as to beat the signs of PMS, which can often involve changes in skin oiliness.

WHEATGRASS

Loaded with vitamins, minerals, amino acids and enzymes, wheatgrass juice can be taken as a drink, applied to the skin or taken as a supplement. As a toner it will fade blemishes and sunspots, stimulate the growth of healthy new skin, and help eliminate toxins.

SUPPLEMENTS CAN SALVE PSORIASIS

Psoriasis, which leaves dry, scaly patches on the skin, can be relieved by taking daily supplements of evening primrose oil, vitamin E and/or cod liver oil to help the skin replenish its moisture levels.

BE A COD LIVER LOVER

Cod liver oil has long been used by women to maintain beautiful skins. It helps to regulate the natural oils in the skin, preventing dryness without making it feel greasy or causing spots and blemishes.

ZAP SPOTS WITH SPIRULINA

Spirulina is a blue-green algae that contains high levels of amino acids and antioxidants, probiotics and phytonutrients – which can be passed on to our bodies to promote healthy skin and hair. Taken as supplements or used as a mask, it is thought to work against blemish formation.

SELECT SELENIUM

The body only needs selenium in tiny amounts but it is crucial for preventing disease, boosting the immune system and helping the skin stay hydrated and undamaged. Selenium protects against toxicity from heavy metals in pollution and works as a healing antioxidant.

E MAY BE WHAT YOU NEED

Vitamin E is perhaps the body's most important antioxidant, which prevents damage from sun, pollution and modern lifestyles caused by free radicals and oxidation. It has been shown to help skin stay young and healthy looking.

PINE FOR PERFECT SKIN

Another of nature's very own antioxidants, utilizing the natural protective enzymes and antioxidants of the French pine tree, pine bark extract is an excellent supplement to maintain skin health.

IMEDEEN FOR AGEING

A natural nutritional supplement containing bio-marine ingredients, vitamin C and zinc, Imedeen nourishes the skin from within to combat the signs of ageing, such as wrinkles, age spots and dry, weak skin.

WISH UPON A STAR

Starflower oil, extracted from the herb borage, is thought to be even more effective than evening primrose oil because of its incredibly high levels of gamma linoleic acid (GLA), an essential ingredient for skin health.

THE GENUINE ARTICHOKE

Artichoke is one of the oldest medicinal plants for detoxifying the skin and body. Artichoke leaf extract, containing a chemical called cynarin, stimulates the production of digestive enzymes to help break down food and encourage the release of toxins.

SPECIAL OCCASIONS

BEAUTY EMERGENCIES

BANISH GREEN WITH KETCHUP

Blonde hair that's been tinged green from the copper and chlorine in swimming pools can be treated with a good dose of tomato ketchup – apply it from the roots to the tips and leave on for ten minutes, then rinse off for instant colour correction.

ESCAPE RED-EYE

Red eyes, especially if they're dry, can be a symptom of low vitamin A. Boost your eye health with betacarotene, found in red, orange and yellow fruit and vegetables. Use 'artificial tears' to ease redness. Eye drops that contain a vasoconstrictor to shrink blood vessels are only a short-term answer and may lead to worsening red eyes.

TEST YOUR IODINE

If you have coarse hair, dry skin and suffer from tiredness, you may be experiencing low iodine levels. Seafood and seaweed are the best sources, or ask your doctor for an iodine test if you're really worried.

DON'T BE A RED-RIMMED SPECTACLE

Lack of vitamin C can lead to styes and inflammation and redness of the rims and whites of the eyes. Rich sources are citrus fruits and juices, kiwis, strawberries, broccoli and potatoes.

COMB AND DRY

If your lashes look more clumpy than naturally dark and luscious, don't wet them in the hope of removing your mascara – the mascara will just clog. Comb through dry lashes with an eyelash comb.

DE-PUFF UNDER-EYE BAGS

If you wake up in the morning with puffy, swollen eyes, apply a gel-based under-eye product to de-puff the tender skin around your eyes, followed by a cool compress – eye masks, which can be kept in the fridge overnight, are a great choice.

SMOOTH A BLOTCHY TAN

There is only one real solution for an unevenly applied fake tan – exfoliate, exfoliate, exfoliate. If you don't have the time to invest, try a tan remove; even if it's not the brand of your fake tan, it should neutralize some of the colour.

POWDER IT OUT

As a quick solution to greasy or oily hair, particularly around the forehead, a dab of translucent powder along the hairline can soak up excess moisture and tide you over until you hit the shower.

HIDE TANNING MISTAKES

If you're out and about in the evening, a light-reflecting product will help even out skin tone and disguise any major streaks caused by badly applied self-tan.

PRIME SKIN WITH POST-LUNCH POWDER

After lunch the skin on your face can often become shiny and greasy. Dust on an oil-free powder to cut out the shine, but don't go overboard; just stick to a thin layer and reapply the powder later if necessary.

ICE THOSE COLD SORES

If you feel the tingling sensation of a cold sore, treat the area with ice immediately, which can help reduce the inflammation around the site and stop the sore from developing. Once the sore has erupted, dab it with salt and lemon.

BIG SQUEEZE

You've squeezed a spot and it's red and inflamed. Now what? Apply antibacterial ointment and wait for the area to dry. Then apply concealer to the red area and over the base of the spot. Avoid covering up a spot with loose powder before it's dry as the powder can cause the spot to turn crusty – wait until the blemish has stopped weeping first.

PENCIL IT IN

To correct over-plucked eyebrows, choose an eyebrow pencil as close to your brow colour as possible and lightly pencil in, following your natural line. Use short pencil strokes, then brush out your brow to soften the line.

TRY THE TOOTHPASTE TRICK

If you suddenly find you have a spot the night before a big party or interview, apply toothpaste to it overnight, which will help dry out the skin and reduce redness around the area.

HAVE A CUPPA FOR PUFFY EYES

For soothing and reducing puffiness in tired, swollen eyes, soak a couple of tea bags in warm water. Squeeze them until just damp and rest for ten minutes with the tea bags on closed eyes. Tea's natural antioxidant properties will get to work on your problem.

TAKE THE SPONGE

If there's one thing you should carry with you in case of beauty emergencies, it's a packet of clean cosmetic sponges, which can be used to smooth out or reapply foundation, blend creased eye shadow and blend streaky areas.

BIG DAY... & NIGHT

BE LAVISH WITH LASHES

Create lush lashes by using an eyelash curler and applying two thin coats of lengthening mascara. Don't overwhelm your lashes with too many coats, especially if your big moment is in the daytime, because your lashes can look clumpy and there's more chance of fall-out. Waterproof mascara is longlasting and won't run if you shed a few tears of joy.

GET A PROFESSIONAL LOOK

Head to your nearest make-up counter or boutique for a special consultation. Not only will they be able to show you great colours, but they'll also give you tips on techniques and insider tricks as well. Sometimes high-profile make-up artists make store visits so keep an eye out for any advertisement giving dates and times for these free events.

TEST WHAT LOOKS BEST

Always try at least one test-run of what you'd like to look like on your big day – with full dress, hair and make-up. Do it a few weeks before the big event and time yourself so that you know to leave enough time on the day itself. For make-up, think about what time of day you want to make your best impression, and don't be afraid to change your look if the occasion runs from day into evening, adding some darker colours or sparkle if you are going to be dancing later on.

AVOID THE BURN

Don't get too much sun before a big event. Sunburns, peeling skin and tan lines can sabotage your special day because they're difficult to cover up completely.

UP-DO HAIR-DO

For a wedding day, black-tie event or other formal occasion, try a sleek sophisticated chignon. Visit your hairdresser for a trial run first to see how it will look and whether it will suit your dress. Your stylist will be able to advise on using hairpieces and aids to achieve the look you want.

KEEP YOUR FACE ON

Give your foundation staying power by using a gel foundation primer before you apply your make-up. Add a light dusting of loose powder to prevent any unwanted shine.

HOLIDAY BLUES

STAY ABOVE THE CUT

Before you go on a beach holiday, take a trip to the hairdresser
for a pre-holiday trim. Damaged ends will only get worse when
exposed to the drying effects of sun, salt and chlorine, so make
sure you set off with your hair in tiptop form.

CARRY ON CAMPING

Space is at a premium in a tent so you won't want to take your
usual bottles of cleanser and toner. Extra-mild baby wipes are
a brilliant substitute, even for removing stubborn mascara, and
can be helpful for many other cleaning tasks.

STROLL IN THE SEA

Give your bum and thighs a workout by strolling in water that's at
least knee deep. It will keep you cool in the sun and, because you're
working against resistance, help tone up your legs and bottom.

CURL AND DYE

Have your lashes curled and dyed before you jet off to the beach
and you won't have to worry about waterproof mascara or panda
eyes. Tints have the added bonus of swelling your lashes, making
them appear thicker.

BE SHORE-FOOTED

Walking on sand is one of the best ways to naturally exfoliate
your feet and reduce foot tension, as the hard grains give you a
massage and pedicure at the same time!

PICTURE PERFECT

FIND AN INTERESTING ANGLE

Look at photos of yourself that you like and try to replicate your
position in the future. Many people look better with their head
slightly angled to the side than straight on.

USE CONTRAST

Photography, especially if there's a flash involved, can wash out pale
colours. To prepare for important photographs, consider putting on a
little more make-up than normal to ensure you look your best.

GO YELLOW IN A FLASH

Foundations with slightly yellow undertones work best with
flash photography, so be careful with rose tones which can look
harsh and make you appear red in the face.

THINGS ARE LOOKING UP

If someone is taking a shot of your face and you want your
cheeks to look slimmer, ask them to take it from above you.
Looking up at the camera will widen your eyes and narrow your
cheeks. A quick trick to avoid the appearance of a double chin is
to touch your tongue to the roof of your mouth.

DON'T BE BROWBEATEN

Remember that photos increase contrast, so don't use dark
shadows or pencils to define your brows, as this may leave you
looking stern rather than stunning. Likewise too much kohl
eyeliner and smoky eyeshadows can create dark pools in the eye
area, making your eyes appear much more deeply set.

SIDE ON

For a slimming standing pose, copy the celebrities and hold your body at a three-quarter pose with one foot in front of the other and with your arms held away from your body – this will minimize the amount of space your body takes up and make your extremities look leaner. Stand tall with the shoulders back. At the moment before the picture is taken, tuck your bottom in slightly – this thrusts the hips out a little and makes your torso look longer.

SEASONAL BEAUTY

LESS IS MORE IN SUMMERTIME

If you change one thing with the seasons, make it your base. Winter foundation will look dull and heavy in the summer, when the light is brighter and your skin is a different colour. Switch to a lighter formula, a tinted moisturizer or just use concealer and a sunscreen.

LIGHTEN YOUR SCENTS

Choose a light formula of fragrance for the summer months – an eau de toilette or a body spritz in the floral or ozonic family is more refreshing and suitable than the autumnal woody and spicy chypre and fougère fragrances.

MASK THE PROBLEM

Once a week during summer, use a face mask derived from fruit to help rebalance and rejuvenate summer skin, removing excess oils without drying. Avocado, cucumber and papaya are all great fruit mask choices.

WAKE UP WITH WATER AND LEMON

This Chinese herbal remedy is a sure-fire method of energizing your body. It will detox your entire system, including the liver and gall bladder, which means your body will be able to clean the blood faster to rid itself of the toxins responsible for poor skin. Simply add a few slices of fresh lemon or the juice of half a lemon to a cup of hot water and drink it.

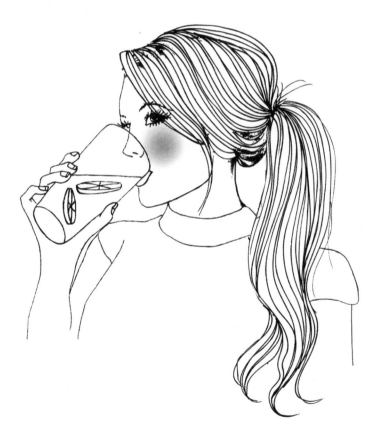

DON'T BE HOT TO TROT

The thought of a long, hot bath on a cold, winter day can be appealing, but over-exposure to hot water can dry skin out even more. Keep baths or showers short, limit them to one per day and use warm, not hot, water.

REMEMBER THE SUN

Even though the sun may no longer be generating high summer heat, don't take that as a sign to throw away your sun block. Dermatologists now recommend an SPF of 15-30 for all skin types in summer, and 15-20 during autumn to prevent sun damage.

GO HOT AND COLD

Start the winter's day with a warm shower but, before you get out, switch to cold water for about 15 seconds, then turn the water from cold to hot and back a few times to stimulate sluggish circulation and to invigorate the skin.

GET RICH QUICK

Use a rich daily moisturizer to keep skin plumped up and well oiled during winter months when it can often become dry and dull. This will help it retain a healthy glow. If possible, avoid AHAs, retinol products and strong exfoliators that strip away your skin in winter and look for enriching ingredients such as vitamin E, amino acids, hyaluronic acid that will quench dry skin.

NO TIME TO CHAP

Chapped lips are often the most noticeable problem when it comes to dryness in the winter. Use a highly moisturizing lip balm, which provides a protective barrier, with vitamin E for good elasticity.

SCRUB UP WELL

Exfoliate once a week to remove dead skin cells and allow the skin to absorb extra moisture, which is lost from the skin's lower layers during winter because of harsher, cooler temperatures. It will help your skin stay pink and glowing rather than grey and dull.

GO MILD

Throw away soap, which can irritate drier skin, and switch to a milder, gentler cleanser for face and body. Soap can irritate and exacerbate dry skin conditions. Instead of rubbing yourself dry, pat to remove excess moisture.

TAKE MATTERS IN HAND

Pay extra attention to hands and feet in winter, when skin can crack and peel. Always apply hand cream after you wash your hands and limit exposure to water by wearing rubber gloves for washing up and cleaning.

TRAVEL

BE A WATER BABY

For every hour onboard a flight, you can lose 100 ml (3½ fl oz) of water from your skin. Keep hydrated by drinking at least 250 ml (8½ fl oz) of water every hour and moisturize your face and body well before flying.

MILK IT UP

Taking a supplement of milk thistle if you're travelling abroad will help aid digestion, protect against stomach bugs, boost your immune system and help your liver deal with holiday excess.

TRAVEL WITH A TINT

Tinted moisturizer is an excellent product for travelling. Not only is it easy to transport and apply, but it can work equally well as a moisturizer, foundation and SPF all in one. It's also less drying than many foundations, which is a must for dehydrated skin.

SLEEP IN THE CLOUDS

The best thing you can do on a plane is to sleep as much as you can. Get comfortable by using a neck pillow, as this area of the body is the one most prone to stiffness after a flight. Invest in an eye mask and ear plugs to block out excess light and noise, whatever the distractions.

USE A FACE TREATMENT

Instead of accepting that flying will make your skin look bad, fight off dullness by using a face treatment while you're on board, particularly on your cheeks, which are often the first areas to show telltale signs of dehydration like fine lines.

MULTITASK YOUR MAKE-UP

Triple crayons and multi-use products like lip and cheek stains are great for travelling because you can apply them on the go with fingers for a quick boost and they take up precious little space in your handbag. Vaseline also makes a great moisturizer, lip balm, highlighter and first-aid salve.

GLOSS IT UP

If you're travelling to warmer climes, lipstick sometimes seems too chalky or heavy. Instead, take a lipliner and lip gloss in your handbag. Line lightly or colour in the whole lip for an instant natural boost that will stay on your lips for hours.

USE UP YOUR FREEBIES

Take any extra free trial-size products from magazines or beauty counters with you. Don't be afraid to ask for samples at beauty counters – in addition to providing good miniature-sizes for travelling and weekends away, it will enable you to try out a product first before investing in a costly purchase for the full-size item.

FLEX THE FEET

For a quick exercise during a train, car or plane journey where you will be stationary for some time, stand on one foot and bend the other behind you, grasping the ankle in your hand. Now flex and unflex your foot – this will keep the blood flowing and help prevent thrombosis and pins and needles.

DON'T TOIL WITH YOUR TOILETRIES

Decant your everyday supplies into plastic bottles to take with you – this will avoid any glass breakages and ensure that your toiletry kit is user-friendly and lightweight.

CLEANSE WITH CLOTHS

Always pack cleansing cloths for a long flight, which will help you keep skin clean and clog-free throughout your journey. Follow with moisturizer to prevent the skin from drying out, and you'll arrive looking as bright-faced as ever.

VANITY CASE

Keep everything at home that you can, taking only the essentials with you. Look for multiple-use products, such as cleansers that double as moisturizers, body lotions that are also formulated for hair conditioning and shea butter balm that conditions nails, hands and lips. A palette of lip, eye and cheek colours will take up much less space than individual products.

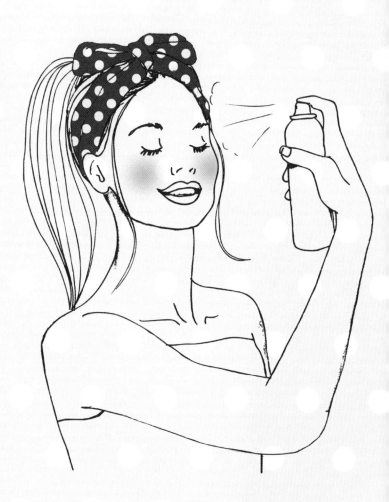

WAKE YOURSELF UP

Humidity is usually less than 20 per cent in airplanes. To freshen dehydrated skin and eyes on longhaul flights, splash your face with cold water and apply plenty of light, non-clogging moisturizer and an eye cream. This will tone the skin and enliven puffy eyes. Spritzing the face with a rosewater atomizer during the flight will also help keep skin supple and soft.

BE BOLD WITH BRONZER

Travelling often makes skin look tired and dull. Bronzer is a great all-round product for warming up pale skin and gives you a glow. It can also be used as a blush or eyeshadow for a more grown-up look.

BRIGHTEN UP

To instantly enliven a tired face, blend a bit of illuminizer or radiance booster over the centre of the chin, the bridge of the nose and the middle of the forehead, which will help give the appearance of a natural, vital glow. If your neck or shoulders are bare, add a little there, too.

YUMMY MUMMIES

BANISH BRUISES WITH MARIGOLD

Pregnant skin is more prone to bruising. Make a bruise-busting infusion with a handful of marigold (calendula officianalis) flowers and 300 ml (½ pint) of boiled water. Steep for five minutes, allow to cool, then wipe the bruised area. Arnica cream is a good homeopathic alternative.

CHOOSE CREAM CAREFULLY

The best creams to prevent stretch marks from occurring are those that contain collagen and elastin, which help regenerate the skin's lower layers and reduce the chances of it being stretched and scarred.

FEED HUNGRY SKIN

The turnover of skin cells is accelerated during pregnancy as the metabolic rate increases, so make sure you nourish and moisturize more than normal to keep skin looking healthy. Concentrate on areas that expand, like the breasts and abdomen. Choose moisturizers that are as pure as possible, such as cocoa butter, as everything you put on your skin has a chance of being absorbed into the bloodstream.

E-RASE STRETCH MARKS

Use vitamin E cream on stretch marks, massaging it into delicate or affected areas once or twice a day to make them less visible and to prevent others appearing in the first place.

BE PATIENT WITH PIGMENT CHANGES

Some women suffer marked pigment changes on their face in pregnancy – called chloasma – because of hormonal changes. If you suffer from this, avoid the sun (which makes it worse) and use make-up to even out your skin tone. Your complexion should revert to normal a few months after the baby is born.

SWIM WELL AS YOU SWELL

Swimming is one of the best exercises for pregnancy because all the body is supported, but chlorine and chemicals can strip skin of moisture and leave it feeling dull and dry. Make sure you use rich body lotions to counteract the drying effects.

STAND TALL

With all the changes in weight and gravity that your body goes through as part of a normal pregnancy, your back may tend to slouch. Try to keep your hips in line with your shoulders rather than pushing them forward as you stand or walk. Good posture will not only help you look taller and less dumpy but will evenly distribute the strain of the added baby weight.

FAKE TAN MAKES MARKS FAINT

Fake tan will help conceal stretch marks by colouring the skin and minimizing their visibility. This trick is especially good for silvery pink marks. Real tanning, however, makes stretchmarks more obvious, so stay out of the sun.

CHANGE PRODUCTS

When you're pregnant, hormones cause changes and sensitivity in your natural skin and hair, so reconsider the suitability of your normal products, which may not be the best to use at this time.

LOVE YOUR CURVES

Instead of worrying about your growing curves, make the most of them with softer hair and make-up for a more feminine look. It's only nine months, after all, and the sooner you accept your new curves, the more you'll enjoy them!

FEED YOUR FEET

Feet can get tired and swollen in pregnancy as the body copes with high levels of blood and fluid circulating in the body. A refreshing foot gel with menthol will really pep you up at the end of a long day, especially if you rest with your feet up.

RETREAT FROM RETIN-A

Increased androgen levels make women more prone to blemishes during the first three months of pregnancy, but you should avoid using acne medications which may cause harm to the developing foetus. These include vitamin A-derivative lotions such as Accutane and Retin-A.

DON'T REACH OILING POINT

If your skin suffers from oiliness during pregnancy, particularly on your face, make sure your cleansers, moisturizers and suncreams are labelled as non-comedogenic (not pore-blocking) and non-acnegenic (not spot-causing).

EXTEND YOUR EXFOLIATION

Skin regenerates itself more quickly during pregnancy, which means dead skin cells are more likely to build up on the surface, causing dullness and spots. Thoroughly cleanse your face morning and night and use a gentle exfoliator on the face and body two or three times a week to keep skin soft, clear and uncongested.

EXTREMITIES NEED EXTRA CARE

Skin on the hands, feet, lower legs and arms is often neglected by the circulation system during pregnancy, as the body concentrates on the growing baby. Gentle exercises and massage can help encourage blood flow to the area to counteract dryness and tingling sensations.

FACE UP TO THE NEW YOU

Many women's face shapes change during pregnancy, becoming fuller and more rounded. Rather than lamenting it, ask your hairdresser to suggest subtle changes to your hair to flatter your new look – straight, shoulder-length hair can help slim cheeks, for example.

CUT DOWN ON CHEMICALS

Instead of using chemical products or straighteners to create a smooth look, which might affect the baby, dry your hair straight using a straightening balm, a natural bristle brush and a nozzled hairdryer. Alternatively, try a light-hold gel to keep natural curls tamed.

BABY KNOWS BEST

Mild baby products are suitable for sensitive skin that is going through hormonal upheavals, so raid your child's supply of baby oil, shampoo and talcum powder. Choose unscented varieties.

COUNT TO THREE

Most doctors and hair stylists recommend not submitting your hair to any chemical processes during the first three months of pregnancy because of extra sensitivity to chemical fumes. This includes colouring, perming or chemical straightening. Even after this, always seek professional advice, as there is ongoing debate as to whether the processes are safe for the baby. To make safe hair colour changes, try a hair wand, gel or mascara, which give a temporary non-toxic colour highlight that only lasts as long as your next wash.

IT MAKES SCENTS

Make the most of your heightened sense of smell and give yourself a lift by spritzing on a clean, fresh scent. Choose a light floral or ozonic fragrance that won't overpower you or make you feel nauseous.

GO VEGGIE

Any hair colouring process should avoid touching the skin and scalp to prevent the absorption of chemicals into the bloodstream during pregnancy. To be safe, opt for highlights and streaks which do not touch the scalp, instead of all-over colour. Rather than your usual bleach or ammonia highlights while pregnant, ask for vegetable dyes or use henna, which do not contain chemicals.

IT'S HARD NOT TO DRY

Breastfeeding can make hair very dry, as the body directs most of its nutrients towards the baby. It should return to normal once you stop, but an extra-moisturizing shampoo and deep conditioner will help until then.

MASSAGE YOUR BUMP

Skin is under a great deal of pressure during pregnancy, with a lot of stretching to do, especially in the abdominal area. Massaging your bump with oil, cream or gel will keep skin supple and elastic, and boost circulation. This will also provide relief if you suffer from an itchy belly.

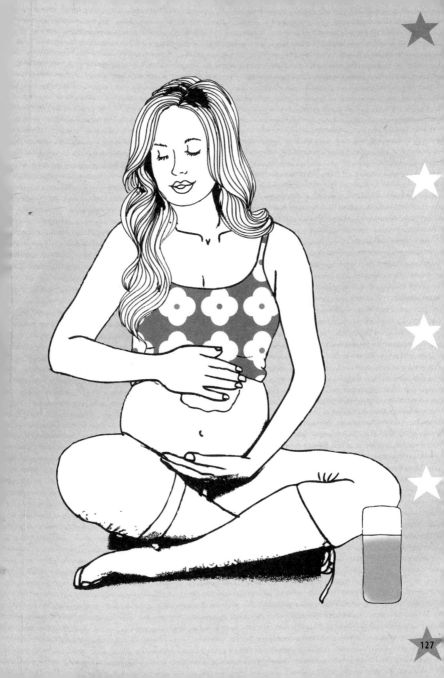

INDEX